TEEN WORLD
WORLD
Confidential

TEEN WORLD Confidential

Five-Minute Topics to Open Conversation
About Sex and Relationships

Kim Cook, RN, CHES

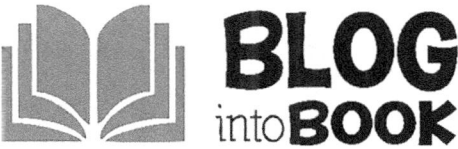

Published by Blog Into Book
3971 Hoover Rd. Suite 77
Columbus, OH 43123-2839
www.GatekeeperPress.com

Cover Photo of Author by Donna Bode.

ISBN: 9781619846067
eISBN: 9781619846074

Printed in the United States of America

Dedication

This book is dedicated to my three daughters—because, as my youngest explained, it only makes sense to dedicate a book to one's children. She is correct. Jenny, Caitie, and Molly, you are the sunshine in my world and the reason for my being. I thank God for you every. single. day.

I also dedicate this book to young people, parents, and other caring adults who are seeking honest information to complicated concerns about sex and relationships, and to the educators and healthcare providers who offer this support and knowledge.

Contents

PERSONAL SAFETY:
you can't hold their hand forever 74

MEDICALLY SPEAKING:
outsourcing medical knowledge....................................... 114

CONTRACEPTION:
how to prevent early grandparenthood 164

SEXUALLY TRANSMITTED INFECTIONS (STIs):
hazardous conditions ahead 194

PARENT SUPPORT:

ADDITIONAL RESOURCES:

DISCLAIMER

ACKNOWLEDGMENTS

Introduction

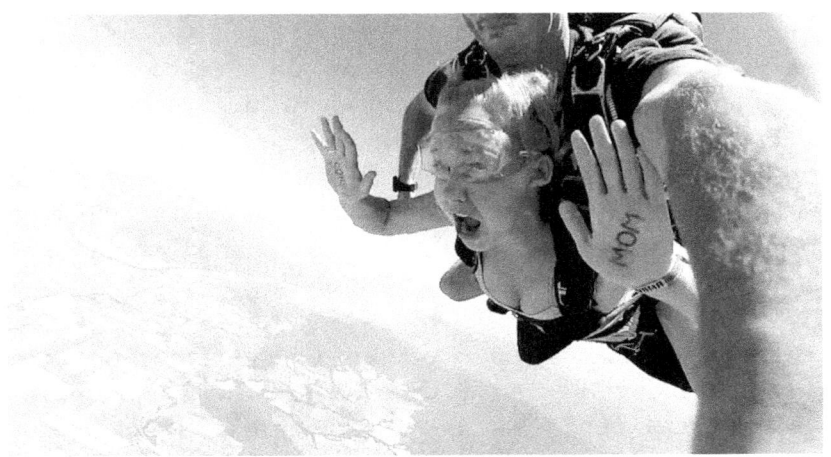

As parents you do your best to give your children guidance and advice ("If I catch you drinking you are grounded!!!") to help them become the amazing humans you know they are capable of becoming. (After all, they are *your* kids…)

My youngest daughter studied abroad in Australia. What a great experience, right? For spring break, she asked my husband and I if we'd mind if she joined an adventure trip with some of her friends. "Sure!" I said…. "just no scuba diving, bungee-jumping, or skydiving." (Did I mention this was an *adventure* tour?). She agreed. Kind of. I think what she said was, "Oh, Mom. You don't need to worry about me!" About two weeks later she sent me this photo. If you look carefully you'll see that the writing on her hands reads, "SORRY MOM."

Parents want the best for their children. We want them to grow up to be healthy, productive members of society, and happy in their future romantic relationships. You also want them alive. Fortunately, Molly survived her jump….and she plans to do more. (Are you *kidding* me??!!) As your children evolve and become their own persons, you learn very quickly that sometimes you gotta let 'em go in order for them to figure out their place in this world.

As your children get older, not only do they become more adventurous, but they become more and more aware of their emerging sexuality. In fact, sexuality becomes an integral part of their teen years, thanks to those abundant hormones. It is your responsibility as parents to help your kids navigate these important years of change and to answer their questions honestly and without judgment.

The more information you have access to and the more open you are when talking with your kids, the easier these conversations will become. Some young people are more willing to talk about this stuff with people other than their parents/caregivers, and that is okay. It's not you—it's them. Well, okay, maybe it is you, too. Once you find a comfortable balance with these conversations, they become easier. Have your child take the lead…you will get a pretty good idea where they are coming from.

If you look closely at the photo again, you will notice that my daughter, Molly, is jumping in tandem with an "expert" jumper. (Seriously?? Is he *really* an expert? Where are his "expert" papers? I need *proof*!!) Parents, teachers, and caregivers are that "expert" who attaches to your precious children to help them make their "jump" into adulthood. You can help push them out the proverbial door with the information and tools they need to make a (relatively) soft (and sometimes bumpy) landing.

Teen World Confidential offers parents and other caring adults tips and tools to inspire medically accurate, honest conversation between you and your mini-me. Information is presented in fast-paced five minute reads that fit into your busy schedule. Killing time waiting in the car for your kids to finish practice? Pick up *Teen World Confidential*, open a random page, and gain fresh insight about current issues affecting teens, 'tweens, and families. Explore conversation starters–and roadblocks–that can open the door to honest communication that will continue through the teen years.

Over the last three years, students have shared with me, anonymously, concerns and questions they have about sex. These quotes will introduce topics discussed in this book. Questions such as, "Why aren't parents more open with their kids about sex?" and "How do you tell your parents you are not a virgin?" These are very real concerns young people have. They want to talk to you. In fact, in an informal poll, I found that parents, not peers, were the primary influencers for teens when making sexual health decisions. *The National Campaign to Prevent Teen and Unplanned Pregnancy[1]* found this to be true as well.

Sexual health is not only about penises and vaginas, birth control, and sexually transmitted infections (STIs). It encompasses so much more. Decision-making, healthy relationships, values, responsibility, and respecting others are the necessary foundations your child requires as they navigate their blossoming sexuality.

My experience as a birth control educator, maternity nurse, middle and high school health teacher, elementary school nurse, and certified health education specialist (CHES) affords me the academic background necessary to educate and inform parents and other adults about such an important topic. However, my most important role, that as the mother of three grown daughters, has

---

1   https://thenationalcampaign.org/resource/survey-says-october-2016

given me the personal experience that allows me to be empathetic and genuine when talking to parents about sex. I get it. There are no easy answers. Only you know your child and the best approach to take with them. However *Teen World Confidential* offers information that allows parents to be informed, enlightened, and oh, yes, cool. Well, sorta.

TeenWorldConfidential.com, an online resource for parents about adolescent sexual health, was birthed from my idea that perhaps it's the parents who need sex ed resources. After all, parents are their child's first sex educators, and educators must be knowledgeable.

Grab a cup of coffee or a glass of wine and dig in to the sometimes humorous and always informative collection of the most popular blog posts featured on the *Teen World Confidential* website.

"How do you tell your parents you are not a virgin?" Female, 11th grade

"How do you tell your parents you are not a virgin?" Female, 11th grade

"Why is there so much stigma about it?" Female, 12th grade

"Is it weird to be scared of having sex?" Male, 11th grade

"I feel like adults talk so much about the dangers of sex that some people are scared of it." Female, 12th grade

"Why is it bad?" Male, 12th grade

COMMUNICATION:

**how to pretend to be a sex-pert
without freaking your kids out**

Using the Barrier Method when Talking to Kids about Sex

Research has repeatedly proven that when parents talk honestly and openly about sex with their children, they are more likely to wait before engaging in sex for the first time and more likely to use protection. In other words, adolescents are actually listening to their parents.

A recent study by Laura Widman and colleagues (Parent-Adolescent Sexual Communication and Adolescent Safer Sex Behavior: A Meta-Analysis) notes that conversations between teens and mothers encourages safer sex practices, even more than conversations between fathers and their children.[2] It is noted in Widman's study that daughters tend to have more frequent sexuality-based conversations with parents–usually their mother–than sons do. Because of these conversations, daughters are more likely to use protection.

Sue, a mother of three states:

> *"I never had a real sit-down, scheduled talk. It was more casual when things popped up. None of my kids really dated in high school so there was never the talk that occurred out of necessity. My parents never had that talk with me and I'm ashamed to say I followed suit. My husband would never speak about it because in his mind premarital sex was wrong and they just shouldn't do it. I took opportunities when conversation went that route to instill bits of wisdom. My main concern with them was that they would always be open with me and ask questions."*

A study by Ellen Wilson and colleagues called "Parents' Perspectives

---

2   Widman L, Choukas-Bradley S, Noar SM, Nesi J, Garrett K. Parent-Adolescent Sexual Communication and Adolescent Safer Sex BehaviorA Meta-Analysis. *JAMA Pediatr.* 2016;170(1):52-61. doi:10.1001/jamapediatrics.2015.2731

on Talking to Preteenage Children About Sex" noted that fathers are more comfortable answering questions "directly and honestly" about sexuality when approached by their children.[3] Dads report feeling more comfortable talking to their kids about sex. However, they are not typically the parent who purposefully initiates such conversations with the children. It is time to draw fathers into the discussion and encourage men and boys to talk openly and honestly with each other.

Melissa, a mother of three grown children reflects on her experience as her children's educator:

> *"I know that we bought a book and read it with each child. I'm sure I did the majority with all three children because I was around. It was as simple as that. I was home at the appropriate time, during the teachable moments. In subsequent years, I have had much more detailed conversations with my daughters, but would have been mortified to talk to my son. (I'm sure he would have been, too). I asked my husband recently if he had ever had an in-depth conversation with our son about sex and he said no. Obviously, our son figured it out; he and his wife are now expecting."*

Jennifer writes:

> *"I really don't remember any ONE sex talk with my daughter. It was a combination of small conversations, mostly in the car. That seemed to always be a great time for conversations she deemed uncomfortable. The numerous small conversations worked well for me because she always absorbed "parental information" and guidance best in small chunks."*

---

3   https://www.guttmacher.org/sites/default/files/pdfs/pubs/psrh/full/4205610.pdf (2010) Parents' Perspectives on Talking to Preteenage Children About Sex

She goes on to say…

> *"I do remember exactly, however, our conversation (in 3rd grade) about how 'babies are born.' 'Mom, I don't want know how the babies come out (we had already talked about that), but I want to know how they get in there! Don't tell me a stork; that's ridiculous!'"*

Conversational Barriers

According to Wilson's study, **moms and dads** may feel uncomfortable talking to their kids about sex for several reasons. In fact, about a quarter of adolescents have not talked to their parents at all about this impactful topic.

Parents may feel they do not have enough information to provide adequate education for their child or will be asked a question to which they do not know the answer. No worries. There are many resources to help parents educate themselves.

Parents may feel their child is not ready to learn about such topics because they have not shown interest in romantic relationships.

Discussions should be instigated early and often, not just when dating becomes an issue. It is best to help your child be prepared for the mental/emotional, social, as well as physical factors that go into having a healthy relationship. It is difficult to teach that in one afternoon.

Parents may feel they are intruding on a private aspect of their child's life.

There is a difference between being nosy and being interested. Recognizing that your child has romantic interests is not intrusive. In fact, I am willing to bet it is going on right in front of your nose, therefore inviting conversation. I used to send my youngest daughter down to the basement to "distract" my oldest daughter and her boyfriend from any unwanted activity that might be going on. Yes, that is intrusive. I offer no apologies.

Parents may not want to know their child is romantically involved with someone.

Sometimes we do not want to know if our child is sexually active. It is just one more thing we have to deal with as busy parents. I get it. However, I recommend engaging in safer sex conversation now, rather than risking a pregnancy or STI conversation later. You are probably losing sleep worrying about it anyway. Just talk it out and get it in the open.

Parents often struggle with not knowing how to start the conversation or not knowing what to say.

What do you say to get the conversation going? How do you say it without feeling … awkward? Possibly the best solution is to accept the fact that it may indeed *be* awkward. It is what it is. Take a deep breath and just start the conversation.

As illustrated by Melissa, Jennifer, and Sue, using age-appropriate books to instigate conversation, finding a comfortable space to talk, and being open and available to conversation are techniques that parents find helpful when talking to their children about sex. Using media and current events to instigate conversation can be helpful. If your children are younger, start talking now. It will help make conversation less awkward when they are older.

You are not expected to know everything there is to know about sex. Besides, as you have discovered, your child does not think you know anything anyway, so the knowledge you do have will impress and surprise them. However, there are many books and online resources that can provide parents with up-to-date, medically-accurate information. Here are a few to get you started:

Online Resources:
Planned Parenthood
ANSWER
Kids in The House
Office of Adolescent Health
WomanCare Global
TeenWorldConfidential

Books:

- 30 Days of Sex Talks: Empowering Your Child with Knowledge of Sexual Intimacy (Volumes 1, 2, and 3) by Educate and Empower Kids
- It's Not the Stork!: A Book About Girls, Boys, Babies, Bodies, Families and Friends (The Family Library) by Robie Harris
- Being a Teen: Everything Teen Girls & Boys Should Know About Relationships, Sex, Love, Health, Identity & More by Jane Fonda
- Prepping Parents for Puberty Talks: A Compilation of Over 500 Questions Children Ask with Child-Friendly Answers by Lori Reichel, PhD

Children appreciate when parents are engaged and invested in their future. They respond positively to the connection they feel with their parent, especially when talking about sexuality honestly and without judgment. Mothers and fathers have a responsibility to get the conversation rolling. No, you do not have all the answers. Yes, it may be awkward. But honestly, this is a moment to connect with your child on a different level. Not only will they appreciate your effort, but it will inspire them to think twice when making decisions about having sex. Finally, it will give them a memory to chuckle about when they become parents and have to face this issue as well.

It's Not Funny—Or is it? Using Humor to Tackle the Talk

Talking to kids about sex. Yikes.

Any parent who has initiated "the talk" with their child has experienced qualms about what to say, when to say it, and how to say it. It would be awesome to channel a sex-pert during these talks and merely let the words flow succinctly, accurately, and in a manner that eliminates the inevitable eyeball roll of your all-knowing child.

When discussing sexuality with young people, a serious approach is often encouraged as a means to demand respect for the topic. I totally get that. Sexual health is a serious issue that encompasses discussions about decision-making, goal-setting, personal values, healthy relationships–oh, and condoms and sexually transmitted infections (STIs), as well. The information young people learn from their parents, community, schools, religious community, and the media will influence the choices they make now and in the future.

**You ask, "Adolescent sexuality is not funny!
Why humor?"**

Infusing humor into a conversation can increase the comfort level to help engage our kids in meaningful dialogue. A certain levity encourages kids to open up and feel safe asking questions.

Humor evens the conversational playing field. With humor, there is a middle ground in which mutual respect and a commonality can be reached. This can enable two-way, honest conversation. On the flipside, lecturing about the sins of sex automatically turns on the mute button in our child's mind. Remember, they are inundated with s-e-x on a daily basis. Between their own hormones egging them on, media encouraging promiscuous behavior, and peer influences, they grapple with confusing messages. Do not squelch their concerns with an unbalanced lecture.

Infusing humor into the discussion reflects the idea that sex is actually...fun. I know, you are thinking-I don't want my kids to think this is FUN!! Let me throw it back to you–why not?? They will spend many more years having sex than not having sex. Hopefully. Certainly you wish for them to have a fulfilling, satisfying, close relationship with their life partner, right? Sharing a few romantic laughs allows for an intimacy that can only strengthen relationship bonds.

There are a few things to consider when talking to kids about sex with a humorous approach.

1. Be yourself. If you tend to have a zero sense of humor, yet still try to crack a few jokes, your kids will think you have lost your mind. Stay sane.
2. If it is not funny to the child, it is not funny.
3. Not every topic about sexuality should be taken lightly. Dating mishaps? Funny. Dating violence? Not funny.
4. If a child comes to you with a serious question, do not minimize their feelings with a joke and an off-hand comment. Look them in the eye, listen to what they are saying, confirm what they are communicating, then answer the question or merely listen respectfully.
5. Each child is unique, with diverse thoughts about sexuality. The conversational style needs to be custom-tailored to the child.
6. Again–keep in mind there is a time and a place for humor.

Talking to your child about sex may seem daunting initially. It would be convenient to have a one-size-fits-all approach to talk with kids about serious topics such as sex. However, we need to appreciate each child as an individual and approach them in a manner that is comfortable for them. Know your child and adapt to their particular personality. You may have one kid who is all over it and asks detailed questions and another kid who covers their ears in horror.

Fortunately, "the talk" is a misnomer. It is actually a series of talks over the course of their childhood, which allows for many opportunities to share a few laughs about sex. As parents, we have to do the work to enable effective communication throughout the years, but we do not have to do it alone. Use the resources and expertise of parents who have traveled to the dark side and come out of it only slightly scathed.

It is a hell of a lot of work birthing, nursing, nurturing, loving, teaching, and launching our kids, not to mention the money we invest! We want them to grow up healthy, happy, and well-adjusted. After all, we do want them to return the favor when we enter the adult-diaper years. So, lighten up! Sex is a normal part of life. It's okay to take a humorous approach to help open lines of communication. Their sex life depends on you. (Wink.)

Birds and Bees Aren't the Only Ones Who Do It: History of Sex Ed in the United States

I was fortunate to enjoy a visit with my daughter in the quirky, vibrant, exuberant, and lovely cities of Berkeley and San Francisco recently. While in Berkeley, I decided to pop into the Doe Library on the campus of UC Berkeley and peruse the detailed exhibit entitled "Birds Do It, Bees Do It." It is a fascinating collection of sexuality education materials dating back as far as the early 1900s. These artifacts include books, posters, magazines, ads, condoms, and even entertaining video.

There were two displays that most fascinated me. One was an issue of *TIME* magazine from 1971, the other an issue of *LIFE* magazine from 1969. Both covers show young people with looks of confusion, sadness, and maybe even a little fear on their faces. Each cover, despite the obvious difference in the ages of the young people, reflect a sense of innocence.

The cover of *LIFE* states, "The Debate Splits the Nation's Schools." Seriously??? 45 years have passed since these magazines were published and we are still debating the issue of what to teach young people about sex ed in our schools?

Interestingly, conversation surrounding the education of our youth about sexual health actually started in 1940—when the U.S. Public Health Service pressed schools to teach sexuality education—stating it was an "urgent need."[4] That was 75 years ago. And where are we now? The U.S. has one of the highest rates of teen pregnancy in

---

4   http://connection.ebscohost.com/education/sex-education-schools/history-sex-education (2016) History of Sex Education

the western world with 77% being unplanned.[5] Half of the new STI diagnoses are found in young adults aged 15-24. Need I say more?[6]

So what needs to change? Education. Conversation. Removing stigma. Understanding. Acceptance.

As adults, it is our responsibility to discuss the realities about sex with our young people. And by realities, I mean all of it. The risks: emotional, physical, and social. But also, the beautiful aspect of sex: emotional, physical, and social. If you share the good stuff with young people, logic tells us they will likely respect our opinions and advice when we discuss the risks of unprotected sex and the importance of sexual decision-making skills.

I would love to see faces that represent our youth reflect confidence, contentment, and hopefulness rather than the doleful appearance of the youth seen on the covers of *LIFE* and *TIME* magazine all those year ago, wouldn't you?

---

5   http://www.hhs.gov/ash/oah/adolescent-health-topics/reproductive-health/teen-pregnancy/trends.html (2016) Trends in Teen Pregnancy and Childbearing

6   http://www.cdc.gov/healthyyouth/sexualbehaviors/ (2016) Sexual Risk Behaviors: HIV, STD, & Teen Pregnancy Prevention

Stats and Facts:
How Many Teens are Having Sex?

Why is it so important we talk to our kids about sexual health? After all, you *did* tell them to wait until they were married, right? Or in love? Or at *least* in college….? And we know if you told them to wait, they most certainly will! (Shall I remind you of my little skydiving story?)

The fact is, kids are deciding to engage in sexual activity before they are married. Or in college. Or even in love. Don't believe it?

According to The Youth Risk Behavior Surveillance (YRBS)** 2015, 41.2% of students have had sex, compared to 46.8% just two years ago.[7]

** *The Youth Risk Behavior Surveillance (YRBS)* is a survey given to students across the country that asks about different aspects of their healthy (or lack-of) behaviors. The study breaks down results according to gender and race/ethnicity as well, however I used the results for ALL kids. This information is used to look at trends and to figure out if our educational efforts in the community and schools is working. Using that information, we can then figure out the changes needed to improve how we address these health-behavior issues.

Of those:

- 3.9 had sex before the age of 13.
- Only 8.8% used both a condom and birth control at last sex.
- Only 56.9% used a condom at last sex.
- 13.8% used no protection at last sex.
- 6.7% were forced to have sex by the person they were dating.

---

7   http://www.cdc.gov/mmwr/volumes/65/ss/pdfs/ss6509.pdf..(2016)Sexual Identity, Sex of Sexual Contacts, and Health-Related Behaviors Among Students in Grades 9–12 — United States and Selected Sites, 2015

- 10.6% experienced some kind of dating violence.
- 30.1% were sexually active at the time of the survey.
- 17.7% seriously contemplated suicide.

I'm not showing you these statistics to frighten you, because when you think about it, if less than half of high school students have had sex by graduation, then more than half have not! I am almost 100% certain your child is in the 60% who has not engaged in such activities because, well, you asked him or her not to, right?

Whether or not your child is sexually active *right now* is irrelevant. One day they will be, and we want to arm our children with tools to help them make solid healthy choices.

The good news is that in the last 20 years, high school kids have been choosing to wait to have sex. In 1991, 54.1% of students engaged in sexual activity–in 2015 it was only about 41%. Also, kids are using condoms more frequently as well. Yay.

However, out of 20 million new STI diagnoses, half are found in the 15-24 year old age group. Yikes. I don't know about you, but I want to make sure my kids stay healthy. However, if they do contract an STI, I want to be confident they know how to handle their situation.

Be Available to Talk to Kids About Sex: Just Don't Be Weird

I had the honor and privilege of attending a high school health fair geared towards students. What an awesome idea! By having this event, the messages sent to these young people are: 1) You are important enough for the school to devote an entire day to your health and well-being, and 2) There are numerous resources within the community to support your physical, mental/emotional, social, and academic needs–you are not alone. How awesome is that? Kudos to the teacher for organizing this well-attended event.

Sexual health was addressed with booths manned by community services that support HIV/STI testing (Open Door Clinic), pregnancy testing and services (Fox Valley Pregnancy Services), and teen parenting (Teen Parent Connection). Of course, our booth—Teen World Confidential–is a resource for medically-accurate sexual health information for parents and students. The presence of these organizations communicated to the students that sexual health is an important part of being human, and that the adults in the school care about this aspect of their lives. How cool is that?

While there, I had students answer questions related to sexual health education. One result in particular is worth noting. When asked if they felt comfortable talking about sex with their parents, the overwhelming majority answered "yes!" They stated that having a "good relationship" and "open communication" with their parents opened doors to easy discussion. Some stated that parents began the conversation about sex early in their growth and development, therefore talking to parents now is not such a big deal.

Of course there were those that felt they could not talk about sex with their parents because either it is "weird" or "awkward" to do so, or their parents are just plain "weird." (I can relate–my own kids say certain topics are **weird** to talk to me about! Apparently, I become "over-interested" in learning about their new boyfriends. (Well, duh! Do you blame me?)…But I digress.)

My point is… parents, guardians, educators, youth supporters… keep up the good work and keep the conversation going. If you are an adult who does not know how to start, or you feel **weird** talking about sexuality, try these starters:

- Ask them what they learned in health class.
- Discuss a current news story. That shouldn't be too hard–I don't think a day goes by that there isn't some sex-related news story being broadcast, often addressing the topic of consent.
- When watching TV or a movie together, chances are there will be some scene that will relate to sex–use that!
- Arrange for a specific time to sit and talk together. Let them know the topic in advance, however!

Kids are curious–they want to know stuff. But not just about condoms and STIs–they want to know about the really juicy stuff, too… Relationships. Love. Friendship. Sexual decision-making. Values. Responsibility. Needless to say, it is not a one-time conversation. Just remember to be honest about your feelings, values, and even your knowledge about sex. It is okay to say, "gosh, I'm not sure!" if they ask you a tricky question.

Respecting your child's thoughts, opinions, and questions will encourage repeated conversation. If they announce they are thinking of becoming sexually active, this is *not* the time to say very loudly "OH MY GOSH! YOU ARE TOO YOUNG!!!" (But it is okay if you freak-out a little in your head. I know you can't help it…just don't let on.) Listen to what they have to say–they are talking to you for guidance, advice, information. Do the best you can. Be human. Be honest. Be respectful. Use some humor. It's okay to laugh together! But apparently, being **weird** is out.

According to the small sample of students who answered my question, "Are you comfortable talking to your parent(s) about sex?" 69% think it's really kind of cool to talk about sex with mom and dad.

Just don't be **weird** about it.

Navigating Emerging Sexuality

If you have ever been "forced" to learn something new, such as the basics of social media or blogging, I don't have to tell you how frustrating it can be. Just when you think you've got it figured out, another glitch rears its ugly head and sets you back another hour. With any emerging skill, it is crucial to start from the ground and work your way up, regardless of how much general knowledge a person may have. Understanding the basics of any new competence forms the roots from which your new knowledge will (hopefully) grow. That's how learning works.

Your brain builds upon information it already knows. For example, there is a reason we teach people how to add and subtract before we dive into algebra–without the concepts of basic math, algebra just isn't going to happen. And for some of us, algebra just doesn't happen anyway. (Why *do* they put those little letters in math problems, anyway?)

Think about our adolescents and sexual health. Teaching our children about the basics of reproductive and sexual health provides the essential groundwork from which their knowledge can grow. Knowing proper terms for their va-jay-jays (vaginas) and willies (penises) is a great start. (See what I mean?) I'm not saying never use slang–that's not realistic. After all, don't we all want to Save the Tata's? First, be sure kids know basic and proper terminology, then you can start messing with their heads with the slang. Please use appropriate, non-offending slang. Some words are entirely unacceptable–and you know which words I mean.

Modeling skills related to decision-making, consequences from our choices, respect for others, taking responsibility for actions… you get the idea… helps kids develop into respectable humans.

These skills are all part of a person's sexuality, too. They use this foundation to navigate their decisions about when and with whom to engage in an intimate relationship, how to keep themselves and their partner safe from unintended pregnancy or STIs, and how to honor their partner's sexuality values.

What you do, what you say, what you watch…it all matters. It is important for parents to lay the groundwork about healthy sexuality. No, please don't tell them details about your own sex life. Rather, talk openly about issues you see on the media. When you hear a sex-related term, ask them if they know what it means. If not, you can explain it to them using your personal values–or just give it to them straight! You know your own kid. And if neither of you knows the answer, look it up!

Laying the roots for your kids when it comes to the physical, mental/ emotional, and social aspects of sexual health will allow them to build upon that knowledge and navigate their sexual world in a manner that follows their personal value system.

Will they always make the best choice?

Well, let me ask you…did you? It's okay. Even mistakes help build our knowledge base; and that is how we grow and learn as individuals. Offer support and guidance as your young person navigates through adolescence and the incredible physical and personal growth that occurs. It's not always easy, but it's always worth it.

Talking to your Infant about Sexuality

The notice arrives from the nurse at your child's elementary school. "The Talk" will be held at some point during fifth grade. Your eyes bug out, your heart pounds, sweat beads down your chest (okay, maybe that was a hot flash), and you suddenly have a need for a glass of red. Or white. And friends!

Little thought bubbles begin exploding around your head:

Wait, I want to talk to my child before the school does.
No way do I want to talk to my child about this!

My child knows nothing about this; why now?
Oh my gosh, what does my child already know?!

My partner and I need to approach our child as a team.
I am in charge of meals, let my partner deal with this!

My child isn't old enough for this!
Is my child old enough for this?

Your child is about ten years old, and they are going to learn about puberty. Very, very soon. This begs the question, when IS the best time to begin talking to your child about S-E-X?

First we have to understand what the conversations about sex look like. Whether you realize it or not, you have been talking about sexual health with your child for many years already. Have you discussed values important to your family? Have you shared your ideas on love and relationships? Have you asked your child "What do you want to be when you grow up?" Guess what? That's all part of the package! Values, relationships, decision-making, goal-setting all lay the foundation for a person's sexual health. So, take a deep breath! You have already begun "The Talks" without even realizing it!

Understandably, it is much easier to talk about family and personal values than penises and vaginas. However, there are ways to gently work your way into these more intimate conversations without creating an environment of awkwardness. Yours–not theirs, that is.

- Start at birth. Even though your sweet little infant has no clue what you are talking about, they do understand the affectionate inflection in your voice. As you gently clean their cute little bums during a diaper change, be sure to casually and sweetly use proper terminology. Penis. Vagina. Scrotum. Labia. Anus. "Let's clean your vagina!" It seems really weird, I know, but as you continue to name these body parts, you will become comfortable verbalizing these words and your child will become accustomed to hearing them. These anatomical labels will seem no less awkward to say than patella, humerus, or tibia. Okay…knee, arm, or leg. I know that many professionals feel using only proper terminology is the best approach. I am a bit more laid back about it. As an adult I use slang for certain body parts myself. ("Save the Ta-Ta's," for example.) There is a time and a place for everything. So, if you want to call their penis a "wee-wee" once in a while, that is okay. Just be sure proper terminology is commonly used as well. Once you have normalized conversation about genitalia, you have laid the groundwork for open and honest communication with your child.

  Equally important, your child will possess the appropriate language with which to communicate to a healthcare provider or other professionals if a situation arises in which concise information is needed. Not everyone will define slang terms the same way, but anatomical labels are universal.

- Explain good touch/bad touch with your child. Introduce the concept of personal boundaries. Explain how to honor one's instinct/gut feeling to discern uncomfortable situations. Help your child to understand others have boundaries as well. This conversation can begin to take place very simply during the preschool years. However, as your child grows older, the discussions will grow in complexity. Certainly we do not want our children to become fearful; the objective is to empower your child with intrinsic guidance.

- Answer the questions they ask, not the questions you hear. For example, if they ask what a penis is and your response involves a long discussion on erections (no pun intended), you have probably freaked them out a bit and totally missed what they really wanted to know—whether boys *and* girls have a penis—not what the penis is used for. No need to go into too much detail. If they want to know more, they will pursue the line of questioning.

- As your child grows and becomes more aware of the world around them, especially with media being so open, there will be opportunities to discuss deeper sexuality issues such as gender identity, sexual orientation, and sexual activity. Looking for ways to broach certain topics? Listen to their music, watch their TV shows, and offer to drive carpool in which you "innocently" listen in on peer discussions. Use those experiences and topics as openings to engage conversation with your child. However, as Heidi Stevens wrote in a recent article, *Parenting Lessons Gleaned in a Decade*, do not ruin the bonding moment by moaning and lecturing during the program, song, or taxi duty.[8] Just wait and hit them with it later—otherwise you may not be invited into their world again anytime soon.

- As teenagers, you can bet they are becoming quite informed about sex from their peers. The question is, how accurate is the information being shared? I promise, if you bring up the topic of

---

8   http://www.chicagotribune.com/lifestyles/ct-balancing-act-sun-0927-20150923-column.html (2015) After a decade of practice, parenting isn't getting any easier

sex to your adolescent, their ears will not spontaneously combust any more than they will walk out the door to find someone with whom to do the horizontal bop. They are pretty much aware of how they came to be on this earth–by now they know there are no pink or blue storks flying around with bundles hanging from their beaks. The time for honesty and openness is now.

Do not fret.
Rest assured. The program your school nurses are preparing is not as explicit as the students seem to think it will be. You will likely be offered an opportunity to preview the program with other dazed parents. The nurses will be there to answer your questions–and provide medical support if you begin to hyperventilate. Parents typically have the opportunity to "opt out" their child from the program; however, I would advise against that. The other students will have all this great information that they will be giggling about on the school bus. Wouldn't you rather your child learned the facts directly from the nurse rather than second-hand from their peers on the bus?

Yes, jumping into the conversation when your child is ten might feel awkward at first. Trust me on this one–the kids are ready to talk. They are trying to figure out why this particular topic is sooooo important that parents actually have to have letters asking for parent approval. They want to know why the boys are separated from the girls. They want to know…what's the big deal? Tell them. After all, the nurses can give the reproductive facts, but only you can instill the values that you hope your child adopts.

No worries though. "The Talk" in school is really just about puberty and the physical, emotional, and social changes they can expect to experience.

They will leave the sex part of the talk up to you. (Wink.)

Body Image and the Preschool Child: Tips for Creating a Positive Home Environment

As parents are well aware, it is common for preteens, both boys and girls, to self-evaluate their appearance. Yet, did you know that preschoolers are already forming ideas about body image that will last a lifetime? In a recent study by **Jennifer** A. **Harriger, et al.** (2010), it was found that children as young as three are already beginning to understand that "thin" is the ideal which society values as attractive.[9] This requires adults to take a step back and evaluate the messages we inadvertently send to our children. After all, our goal as parents is to create an environment in which a healthy body image can be developed.

There are some simple strategies to help promote healthy body image in our little ones. Try incorporating a few of these suggestions each day as you interact with your child.

Successes: Praise your child's efforts rather than their accomplishments. This reward system is becoming commonly encouraged among educators and parents. Rewarding effort encourages children to work to the best of their ability, therefore developing mastery. Rewarding accomplishment is evaluated externally and can prove frustrating when they are not getting the praise they are expecting.

Appearance: Exclaim what a lovely color their dress/shirt is, rather than how attractive they are while wearing the outfit. "That color really brings out the blue in your eyes!"

---

9   Harriger, J.A., Calogero, R.M., Witherington, D.C. et al. Sex Roles (2010) 63: 609. doi:10.1007/s11199-010-9868-1

Values: Flatter your child with compliments regarding their values. For example, notice when they are friendly to their neighbor or help out a friend. Kindness and friendliness are traits that can be encouraged and further developed over the years.

Media: Be aware of the messages the media is sending our children about gender-specific roles and appearance. Little girls are not-so-subtly
reminded to be beautiful princesses. Our little boys are not-so-subtly reminded to be strong superheroes with iron-abs whose mission is to "save" the princesses. Take time to talk about what real males and females are all about. Read this **great essay by Naomi Perks** in which she addresses external influences young boys face.[10]

Mealtime: As a child, I remember a common mealtime mantra was, "Take what you want, eat what you take." Needless to say, my eyes were bigger than my stomach and sometimes I innocently took more than I could eat. Keep in mind that children will eat when they are hungry and will usually stop eating when they have had enough. Encouraging them to eat, even when their little tummies are full, makes it difficult for children to tune in to their internal hunger signals. Instead, wrap up their leftovers and offer it to them for lunch the next day.

Eating habits: Explain to kids about foods they can *always* eat (vegetables, fruit, lean meat, whole grains) and foods they can *sometimes* eat (sugary treats). This will help them continue healthy eating habits as they grow.

Parental influence: When looking in the mirror, avoid self-depreciating comments. You have a little extra "cush in the tush?"

---

10 http://www.parentscanada.com/family-life/are-superheroes-and-video-games-affecting-boys-body-image (2013) Are superheroes and video games affecting boys' body image?

So what? Your child looks at you with love and admiration, not with a mental measuring tape. By embracing your body–whatever form it takes–your child will learn to embrace their own body. Remind them of all the amazing things a body can do.

Of course we have to get real. Yes, our son looks super handsome in his new suit. Yes, our daughter looks beautiful in her cool outfit. A little praise for their appearance on occasion will not hurt them. In fact, we want them to take pride in their appearance as they go through life.

There is a difference between taking pride in appearance and becoming obsessed with the ideal, however. Take a look in the proverbial mirror. Appreciate how our subtle cues influence our children's developing body image. We can cultivate a healthy appreciation of what a "perfect body" truly is–a vessel in which to enjoy life, experience adventure, and impact the world in whatever positive manner we choose.

Kim T. Cook, RN CHES

"Transgender individuals and their sexual insecurity." Male, 11th grade

"I feel as though LGBT education is important. Teach about the genders, sexuality and protection." Non-binary, 10th grade

IDENTITY:

boys, girls, and everyone in between

LGBTQ....Defined

Facebook recognized that not all individuals identify as heterosexual, there are now options for their users when setting up their profile. In fact, many other organizations have followed suit recently.

Options, you ask? How can there be options? Male. Female. What more can there be? Apparently, Facebook offers about 50 options. Well, I read that somewhere anyway. So, curious, I checked it out. Wow–there ARE a lot of options!

It got me thinking…are people familiar with the terminology that many individuals use to identify themselves? Maybe not. Would you like to know? Good! That's what I like to hear–people who are interested in learning new information to help them become educated, open-minded, people of society.

We have heard the term "LGBT", but I'm not so sure people know what each of the letters stand for. I believe people know it is a term related to the gay community, but that is about it. Sometimes you may hear it referred to GLBT.

LGBT:
"L"–Lesbian
"G"–Gay
"B"–Bisexual
"T"–Transgender

Sometimes you may see it written as such:

LGBTQ or LGBTQQ or LGBTQA or LGBTQQAAIP

"Q" – Queer
"Q" – Questioning
"A" – Ally
"A" – Asexual
"I" – Intersex
"P" – Pansexual

Okay. So, what do these terms mean?

Ally: Someone who supports the LGBT community.

Asexual: Not sexually attracted to any sex.

Bisexual: A person of one sex who is attracted romantically/physically to a person of the same sex OR of another sex.

Cisgender: A person's biology matches their gender identity.

Gay: A person of one sex who is attracted romantically and/or physically to a person of the same sex. Generally, the term is used when referring to men who are attracted to men, however this term can be used to include both males and females who are attracted to same-sex individuals.

Gender identity: The person identifies as male, female, neither, or both. Some individuals do not identify as him/her/she/he. Rather, they prefer to be referred to as them/they.

Intersex: More of a medical thing. A person may be born with ambiguous male and female anatomy–external as well as internal. Sometimes it is obvious at birth, other times it is not noticed until puberty, and sometimes a person never knows! There are several medical conditions associated with being intersex, including Turner Syndrome and Klinefelter Syndrome. This has nothing to do with sexual orientation. Other terms for this are Gender X and hermaphrodite.

Lesbian: A woman who is attracted romantically and/or physically to other women.

Non-binary: A person may use this term when they do not identify as either male nor female, but somewhere in between. This is not the same as transgender.

Pansexual: Attracted romantically/physically to a person regardless of their orientation, gender, identity, or anatomy.

Polyamorous: A person has more than one romantic partner.

Queer: Used by those in the LGBT community to describe themselves as being unique. The word 'queer' can sometimes be interpreted as derogatory, so be considerate when using this term.

Questioning: Refers to a person who is exploring their sexual identity, orientation, or gender identity.

Transgender: Transgender refers to individuals who express themselves as the opposite sex from which they were born. This can include cross-dressers, transsexuals, and others.

Transsexual falls under the umbrella term of transgender.

Transsexual is defined as an individual who was born with the outward appearance of one sex, yet inside they feel like the opposite sex (gender identity). The body does not match the psyche. Some individuals may transition by dressing as the person of the opposite sex to express their gender identity. They may also transition by legally changing their gender or name, or merely by changing their name and pronoun within their social or professional circles.

Some individuals who identify as transgender will elect to transition by undergoing surgical and/or hormonal treatment to allow their outward appearance to match how they identify inwardly. This is referred to as sex reassignment surgery. They may also elect to surgically or hormonally transition partially which can be referred to as gender hybrid. The individual may choose not do anything at all. It is a personal choice.

The term transsexual is not used as much as it used to be. In fact, transgender is often used interchangeably. It is best to ask the individual how they would like to be referred. Keep in mind, these terms refer only to gender identity (do they identify as male or female) *not* sexual orientation (whom they are attracted to romantically).

That is a lot to take in. Don't worry, there won't be a quiz on this. It is important to have a general idea of what people are talking about. And yes, it can be confusing. Especially the transgender/transsexual language.

If you want more information, these are great resources:

http://www.glaad.org (Gay and Lesbian Alliance Against Defamation)
http://www.isna.org (Intersex Society of North America)

https://www.gsanetwork.org (Gay Straight Alliance Network)
http://community.pflag.org (Parents, Families, Friends of Lesbians and Gays)
Between XX and XY: Intersexuality and the Myth of Two Sexes by Gerald N. Callahan, Ph.D. (I loved this book!)
(A special thanks to Dr. Sally Conklin from Northern Illinois University for her support and suggestions!)

———————————

Kim T. Cook, RN CHES

"Should sex be thought out?" Female, 9th grade

"How do you know you are ready for sex?" Female, 10th grade

"What if I am in love?" Male, 11th grade

"Does being in love with someone change what the outcome of your sexual experience is?" Female, 11th grade

"What is the worst thing that can happen?" Male, 9th grade

DEFINING SELF:

**how to help your child answer "who am I?"
without the slightest bit of manipulation (wink)**

R–E–S–P–E–C–T

Last night on my flight home from California, I had the privilege of sitting next to an interesting man to whom I explained my plans to write a book for parents about adolescent sexual health. He didn't even bat an eye; in fact, he thought it was a great idea. Most people look at me and say something like, "Why in the world would you want to do something like that?" often followed by a "God bless you." I'm not going to lie–that usually makes me laugh. But, I'll take a blessing whenever I can get it.

Turns out this man, Bill, had some forthcoming parenting advice when it came to his own kids, who are now grown. I asked if he'd mind if I shared his thoughts; I liked his underlying theme–**Respect Yourself.**

He had some basic rules for his daughter's suitors.

- Do not honk your horn and expect my daughter to run out to greet you like a little puppy. She deserves more respect than that. However, if you do choose to honk, you will hear my bark as I request you leave my home.
- Come to the door, shake my hand, and look me in the eyes. Look at me and see the hidden message in my eyes–that if you so much as lay a hand on my beautiful daughter without her permission, you will have me to answer to. And I run very, very fast.

Some basic life "rules" he wanted his son and daughter to abide by:

- Respect yourself and love yourself. Know that you are capable of making good choices and being confident in those choices. You want blue hair? Wear it proudly. (You won't mind if I dye my hair blue, too, will you?)

2. Make choices on *your* terms, not on the terms of your peers, romantic interests, media, and other outside influences that may pressure you. You are the only one that will live with the consequences–and successes! However, I will gladly take the credit when people say "what great kids you have!"

During our conversation, it was clear he wanted his children to be respected by others and also to respect themselves. He felt if that happened, they would be more likely to make choices that are decent and reasonable. We don't expect perfection from the kids–how dull–but nor do we want to form too many wrinkles and gray hair worrying about our kids! What a cool, enlightened dad.

Helping Your Child Identify Their Goals

How many times have you witnessed a young person, just about to head off to college, roll their eyeballs when asked, "What do you plan to major in?" They must be asked that about 600 times from junior year on…until they graduate from college. However, this is a significant question to ask. Think about it…"What do you want to be when you grow up?" is a loaded question.

We aren't just asking them which career path they want to take. We are asking them how are they going to get there. Where do they see themselves as an adult? What kind of person do they hope to become? What are their dreams? Hopes? Desires?

Yet, we don't often verbalize those questions. We should help them think outside the typical "I want to be a fireman" box and into the "Where do I see myself as an adult and how will I get there" box.

Opening up this type of dialog when our children are young makes it much easier to continue the discussion when they are older. Of course, you need to approach it much more simplistically when they are younger. Little comments about being kind to others or showing examples of adults that are positive role models are ways to get their wheels spinning.

As our kids get older, we can start discussing some of their personal goals and how to reach them. Talk about these points:[1]

* Is the goal realistic in relation to their abilities, talents, and interests?
* What are their expectations when setting the goal?
* What steps must they take to reach their goal?

---

1   Weinstein, Estelle. and Efrem Rosen. Teaching About Human Sexuality and Family: A Skills-Based Approach. Belmont: Thomson Wadsworth, 2006. Print.

- Honor and discuss the commitments needed to achieve the goal.
- What would prevent them from reaching that particular goal? What would merely be a stumbling block? Encourage flexibility. How can they re-route their path if it's not working out the way they planned?
- Is it possible there might be other outcomes? How would that effect other goals?
- Most importantly, encourage them to surround themselves with positive people that will help them achieve their goal.

So, what does this have to do with adolescent sexual health? It has been shown that individuals who have goals and plans for their future are less likely to engage in activities that might risk successfully meeting their goals.[2] Does that mean adolescents will never do anything that will ever put them in a risky situation? Um, no. But it does mean they just may wait a little longer or take fewer risks.

Bottom line, discuss your child's future with them. Help them dream, set goals, plan, and did I say dream? Help them keep the "big prize" within their sight. Don't be a pest by constantly nagging them about doing better in school or else "you'll never be a doctor!" Just relax and enjoy the ride with them. They will change their future idea of themselves throughout their lives. It is so exciting to watch! Just be there for them when they need support.

---

2   Weinstein, Estelle, and Efrem Rosen. Teaching About Human Sexuality and Family: A Skills-Based Approach. Belmont: Thomson Wadsworth, 2006. Print.

Purpose: What is Yours?

Talking to our kids about their sexual health can be tricky or even uncomfortable at times. That's okay—perfectly normal; especially as we are talking about penises and vaginas, birth control, or STIs. But we must talk about those topics with them, just as we talk to them about our other body systems and how to care for those "parts" as well. Remember, we were the ones who taught them how to wipe their bottoms. You cannot get much more personal than that!

But talking about sexual health encompasses more than the biology of sex. It also involves emotional, psychological, and decision-making processes as well.

While attending a conference in Baltimore, I had the honor and privilege of listening to Dr. Victor Strecher speak. He is a professor at the University of Michigan School of Public Health. Sadly, he suffered the loss of one of his daughters a few years ago. He used that grief, along with his expertise, to encourage and support others in their life journey—their purpose.

It was an engaging and inspiring talk encouraging individuals to define their purpose. No, I do not mean waking up and realizing that you have four loads of laundry to catch up on—though that certainly *can* be a purpose for your day. But more like, what is your *authentic* purpose. According to Dr. Strecher, this purpose gives you a reason to get up in the morning; it gives you energy in your life. I am certain there are many days you wonder just exactly *what* you are accomplishing sometimes—I've been down that road as well. But you do have a purpose. Take some time to contemplate the things in your life that you feel passionate about…that excite you.

And while you are doing your pondering, how about approaching the young people in your life? Dr. Strecher believes that having a purpose can serve as potential protection against ill health and toxic addictions. Because my focus is on sexual health for young people, it is my thought (totally unscientifically proven, but still...) that if your child feels like they have a reason to get up in the morning and be a part of the world—a reason to look ahead— they are more likely to make well thought-out choices about their health, including their sexual health. After all, they want to make it to adulthood to fulfill their purpose, too. In fact, we frequently talk to our children about goal-setting which is not so different than having a purpose.

So I suggest to you, when you both have time, ask your child:

- Where do you see yourself in 2 years, 4 years, and beyond?
- At this point in your life, what do you feel is your purpose? They will likely need a little guidance with this question.
- What excites you in life? (Girls in bikinis don't count.)
- What steps will you take over the years to fulfill your life's purpose/goals? (And yes, a purpose may morph—they are still trying to figure "life" out. Heck, so am I.)

Your child may say something like, "Moooommmmmm (or Daaaaaaaaaddddddd) I don't knooooowwwwww." They may throw in a "Quit buggin' me!" But deep down they are listening. You can encourage them to write down their thoughts and then arrange a specific time to visit the local coffee shop or ice cream parlor for a planned conversation with you. If they are not caught off guard, they may be more willing to talk.

Another idea is to take a leisurely walk with them. Studies have shown physical activity can encourage bonding and conversation. According to Dr. Jennifer Carter in an article written by Kirsten

Weir entitled *The Exercise Effect*, Dr. Carter's patients tend to relax and share more when they are walking during therapy.[3] It just may work with your young person, too.

Just make sure you take this time to listen to your child. Really listen. It's their time to speak. Use affirming words like, "I hear you say…" so they know you are paying attention to them. I am betting they will open up even more. Try not to let your eyeballs bulge out if they say something unexpected or surprising. Be coooooolllllll…

In the *Child Trends Research Brief* article "Parents Matter: The Role of Parents in Teens' Decisions About Sex" written by Erum Ikramullah, Jennifer Manlove, Carol Cui, and Kristin A. Moore, studies are summarized that show just how important parents are in influencing their kids when it comes to sexual health decisions–even more than peers! They actually listen to adults, but we have to make ourselves available to them.[4]

This is not a "sex" topic per se, but think about it. This can open lines of communication with the young person in your life that can be helpful when you approach other intriguing topics such as relationship decision-making.

To find out more about Dr. Strecher and his work on finding one's purpose, please visit dungbeetle.org. Yes, you heard me. Dung. Beetle. Check it out–there is a reason he uses that name. There is even information to help coach you through defining your own purpose.

(I do want to disclaim any relationship or partnership with Dr. Strecher. I just wanted to share something that I found pretty cool and relate it to my own purpose … adolescent sexual health education.)

---

3   http://www.apa.org/monitor/2011/12/exercise.aspx (2011) The Exercise Effect

4   http://www.parentactionforhealthykids.org/sites/default/files/Child_Trends-2009_11_11_RB_ParentsTeenSex.pdf (2009) Parents Matter: The Role of Parents in Teens' Decisions About Sex

On that note, I believe my next 'purpose' is a chocolate chip cookie….yummmmm.

Perspective: It's All in Your Head

Ping! Off went my text message alert. Group message to my group of friends from Katie.

"What color is this dress?"

I responded: "Oh, that's a very pretty blue and black dress!"

Another friend countered: "White and gold."

I looked at the photo again. Huh? There is absolutely no gold or white. Taking the high road, I just stated it was a lovely dress, and they should buy it. After all, that was why they were asking, right?

Ping! Off went my text message thirty seconds later.

"What color is this dress?" my daughter in Colorado asks. She also messaged her sisters scattered across the country, as well as my husband. Like he would care about a dress.

And, wait–the same dress as my friend Katie? What is going on?

"Blue and black" I replied.

"Gold and white" wrote my husband, who was in the basement.

Apparently, I was outnumbered. Gold and white seemed to be the "winner" according to the rest of my family. Indignant, I grabbed my phone and marched downstairs.

"Really? You call this gold and white?" I demanded of my husband.

"Well, duh, yes" He responded.

I rolled my eyeballs, explained he was color-blind, and noted his daughters' phones were not working properly.

After a number of heated follow-up texts, there were several questions I asked of myself.

What the heck is going on?
And who found this dress?
And who started this viral mind-blower?
And how does one get their tweet to go viral so quickly? Oh, wait–that's another subject.
But more importantly, whose perspective is correct?

Perspective, which is a person's point of view, is one of my favorite words. It is as unique and individual as the hair on our head and the color of our eyes. We want others to acknowledge our perspective, to understand it, and even agree with our perspective; of course our perspective is the correct way of viewing things, right?

Perspective, whether personal or within a community, can inspire fascinating conversations, incite lawmakers, and even ignite world wars. It can also bring people together. Think about the people you choose to be with. You are likely to gravitate towards people with a similar perspective on life, lifestyle, spirituality, and values.

However, respecting others' perspectives is essential in blurring lines of division that are drawn based differences. We must keep in mind that often our perspective is based upon our upbringing, personal experiences, spirituality, culture, and community, to name a few.

Even siblings who grow up together may have different perspectives merely because they have had different experiences that being an oldest, youngest, middle, or "only" bring.

Varying perspectives make for a colorful and vibrant world of interesting people. Teaching our children to embrace and connect with others who have their own unique perspectives will allow them to grow as humans. It will expand their worldview. It may change their own perspective or inspire others to change theirs.

This applies to sexuality health as well. A comprehensive sexual health curriculum will enable our youth to understand, from a medically-accurate position, the perspective of others when it comes to beliefs, sexual orientation, and influences that shape the uniqueness of each of us. This will influence individuals to become less judgmental and more accepting of others.

After all, perspective is in the mind of the beholder; it is not something that is necessarily wrong or right. It just is.

So, back to the dress. According to Gregory Brown and Mitchell Moffit of the innovative AsapScience, the color of the dress is whatever color your mind perceives it to be. Our perspective, whether it is a color or an idea, is individual and should be respected. Keep an open mind to others' perspectives and use it to spark informative, fascinating, and inspiring conversations.

Who knew a blue and black dress could spark so much conversation and fun?

To view this dress and understand the debate, go to YouTube: https://www.youtube.com/watch?v=AskAQwOBvhc

Values...What's Your Perspective??

There has been some controversy about insurance coverage and the responsibility of one's employer to provide birth control for employees. It got me to thinking...about values, actually. How it is important to have them, share them, act on them. But it is also important to respect the values of others as well. Let me explain...

Comprehensive sex education includes discussion about individual values as it relates to decision-making and relationships. (See? Sex ed isn't just about penises and vaginas!) Making prudent decisions is guided by one's values.

Let's take a minute to ponder...what *is* a value? I define it as an idea, belief, and/or consciousness that allows a person to live their authentic life. It is something that a person holds near and dear to them: a belief that cannot be taken away, though it may certainly morph over time.

I'll share some of my values to give you an idea of different kinds of values. They are not necessarily in any order:

- love of family
- belief in maintaining a healthy lifestyle (does an occasional glass of wine count?)
- lasting friendships
- respecting others' opinions while holding onto my own ideals
- taking time to enjoy the simple and not-so-simple pleasures in life
- education and
- quality medical care.

So, what are some of yours? Take a minute to think about it and write them down.

_____

_____

_____

_____

I bet your list looks a lot like mine!

There are decision-making formulas we teach students in health education classes. Within the formula there is an opportunity to recognize and evaluate one's own values in order to make sound decisions. As an educator, I may have different values than my students and their families, so it is up to each family to talk about their own POSITIVE values: cultural, religious, personal, whatever... Schools can teach skills, but parents and caregivers are indispensable when it comes to continuing the dialogue at home.

We all have different values–and that's okay. After all, we come from different ethnic, religious, cultural, geographical backgrounds. In my opinion, the important consideration is to respect others' values and the perspective that goes along with it. "Perspective" is probably one of my favorite words...(besides "summer"!) Sharing a similar perspective with others about a value builds community and offers reassurance that our thinking isn't totally wacky. However, understanding and accepting that people have different perspectives makes for a more harmonious world...as well as some interesting friendly debates!

Therefore, one's own values should be cherished but not forced upon others. If a person chooses to use birth control, or not, that is a personal choice that likely is affected by their religious, cultural, or family value system coupled with their perspective on how their values should be lived. For example, employers who do not believe in contraception have every right not to use contraception as a personal choice based on their values. However, should their employees be unable to obtain contraception of their choice merely because the corporation who employs them feels an obligation to instill their values upon their devoted employees? We all want to be respected and valued for who we are and not be marginalized or penalized for honoring our own values.

So parents, teachers, caregivers, healthcare providers…whomever you are…teaching positive values to those young people you care for is incredibly important. But one value that is also imperative to teach–as well as model–is the ability to respect others' perspective's and appreciate people for the unique and intriguing people they invariably are.

It is Okay to D–E–C–I–D–E

Before we talk about decision-making, let me give you the world's shortest neurology lesson:

The part of the brain that is involved in self-control, reasoning, and decision-making: the **pre-frontal cortex**, does not fully develop until about the mid-20's. This is the part of the brain that says, "This is a really dumb idea. Don't do it."

The **amygdala** within the limbic system (in the middle of your brain) is responsible for emotions. It develops before the prefrontal cortex does. This is the part that says "I'm really angry."

When you add it up, the underdeveloped prefrontal cortex plus the developed amygdala equals lots of strong emotions and not alway a lot of self-control. This can lead to questionable decision-making skills at times. This does not mean adolescents *always* make bad decisions. It merely means they are still physiologically developing and could use a little help learning how to make decisions and control emotions.

Another thought regarding brain development…through childhood and adolescence, the pathways in the brain that develop and stick around are the ones they use. If they don't use them, they sort of disappear. Therefore, encourage your kids to read–or read to them. Encourage learning a foreign language, participating in sports, visiting museums, playing thought-provoking board games, and creative learning opportunities so those pathways in the brain stick around, not the couch-potato pathways.

*(Want to know more? Watch Dr. Sarah-Jayne Blakemore as she gives an interesting **TedTalk** about adolescent brain development called The Mysterious Workings of the Adolescent Brain.)*

Okay, now that we are all brain experts, let's talk about decision-making.

There are formulas we use to teach students in health education classes that show how to make good decisions. It seems odd that formulas would be written about this, much less that a person even needs to be taught how to make good decisions, but learning skills to make wise decisions will assist them as they grow and mature into adulthood. As the brain develops cognitively, it begins to make connections about decisions and the outcomes that follow.

The model frequently used in schools and healthcare facilities is the D-E-C-I-D-E model. This model is used with some variations. Essentially, these are the steps:

D: **Define** the problem.
E: **Explore** the alternatives
C: **Consider** the consequences
I: **Identify** your values
D: **Decide** and take action
E: **Evaluate** the results and make changes

We often go through these steps without even realizing it. Consider a decision you have made lately. How did you come up with your final decision? I am guessing you went through most of these steps without even realizing it.

For our adolescents, however, we may need to provide a little more guidance. Practicing decision-making skills will help get their thought processes wired up. It is easy to start with simple decisions such as nutritional choices, but then eventually move on to heavier issues such as where to attend college, which friends to spend time with, and their sexual health. They can analyze their thoughts about initiating a sexual relationship, using condoms, remaining abstinent, etc. by utilizing the DECIDE model. Encourage the young person in your life to think through different scenarios before they find themselves in certain uncomfortable situations. This helps them rehearse refusal skills as well.

To help your child practice these skills, come up with a potential sticky situation together. Then simply write the D-E-C-I-D-E acronym on a piece of paper. Talk about what each letter–or step—represents, then present them with a scenario. Have them write each step out and ponder actions and consequences.

If your household is like a humming train station and finding time to sit and write stuff out probably won't happen, just have a conversation in the car. Talk through the different steps, then give your adolescent some different scenarios you can think through together. When they are faced with similar situations in 'real life,' they will have a mental tool in which to refer.

Following is a list of pretend scenarios to help your child think through potential sticky situations. Otherwise, talk through decisions or situations they re dealing with right now.

- You have a big test in the morning. However, your favorite band is playing tonight and you were able to obtain free tickets.
- You are riding in a car with friends, when all of a sudden one of them lights up a joint.
- Your boyfriend/girlfriend wants to have sex. However, you don't feel you are ready yet. Yet if you don't, they say they will leave you.
- You and your significant other are sexually active. Your partner does not want to use condoms, even though condoms are the best way to reduce the risk of unplanned pregnancy, STIs, and
- HIV (other than abstinence).

Let's do one together.

D: Define: Have your child define (or identify) the problem.

> *My boyfriend wants to have sex, but I am not ready yet. He says he will leave me if I do not take our relationship to the next step.*

E: Explore: Talk about the different options available. Focus on the better choices.

My options are:

> *1. Talk with him about my feelings.*
> *2. Have sex.*
> *3. Do something that will please him sexually without having intercourse.*
> *4. Break up.*

C: Consider: What are the pros and cons of each option?

1. Talk to him about my feelings.

Pros: If I talk with him about my feelings, he will understand why I do not want to have sex. Respecting my feelings is a sign of a healthy relationship. Cons: He may not care how I feel.

2. Have sex.

Pros: *If I have sex with him, he said he won't break up with me. I do love him.* Cons: *He may eventually break up with me even if we have a sexual relationship. I may be compromising my values. I do not want to get pregnant or contract an STI. I just don't feel ready.*

3. Do something that will please him sexually without having intercourse.

Pros: *Perhaps if we have oral sex I can buy some time. That will make him happy.* Cons: *But isn't oral sex just another way of having sex? I am not comfortable with oral sex.*

4. Break up.

Pros: *If I break up with him, the pressure will be gone.* Cons: *But I love him and want to stay together.*

I: Identify: Talk about your values–what is important to you? Do you value education? Do you value your friendships? Do you value your sports or clubs? Do you value your health? How will your decision affect your value system?

I value my reputation and my education. My self-worth is at stake, as well. I value the relationship I have with my boyfriend, too, but want to be respected for my feelings. If I choose to have sex, I am going against what is important to me. My long-term goals may be affected if I become pregnant or contract an STI.

D: Decide: What is the decision? Act on it.

I'm nervous, but I think I will talk to him. He needs to understand my feelings and I want to understand his perspective, too. I have been taught that having a healthy relationship requires honest communication. If we do not have a healthy relationship, it is not wise for me to have sex when I am not ready. If he continues to pressure me, I will have to break it off.

E: Evaluate: How'd it go? After your decision has played out, evaluate the results. If you don't like the outcome, go back and explore your options and their consequences, and try again!

I am so happy we talked. He explained he was getting a lot of pressure from his friends to have sex, but he cares about me and does not want me do to something I am not comfortable with. I think we respect each other more than ever before. I made a good choice.

Remind the young person in your life that we all make dumb decisions and mistakes. Learning from our mistakes is how we grow as people and how we learn to deal with life's curve balls. We just want our children to have the mental tools to figure out how to make the best decisions they can by thinking things through a little bit.

Five Words of Wisdom for Adolescents: Stolen from the Walls of the Gym

This morning I returned to the gym for the first time in almost three weeks. It was not my choice to miss those 5:15 AM wake up calls; an injury sidelined me. Okay, okay, I could have adapted my moves. But that is beside the point—it was great sleeping in for a change.

I decided to shake it up a bit and experience a new gym this morning with some friends. As I rode the boot camp struggle bus, puffing and grunting my way around the room, I noticed inspirational quotes scattered around the room. The words, intended to inspire clients to return to the torture chamber–I mean gym–resonated with me through an entirely unrelated lens.

Be Awesome Today.

Of course, it is difficult to deny the awesomeness of friends who actually like to work out with me. They are truly awesome people. But what about our kids? When we tell them to be awesome, are we setting expectations too high? Or should we redefine what awesome means? When I read the word awesome, I think "exceptional" "amazing" "spectacular". Perhaps we can communicate to our kids that it is okay to be their own genuine self, flaws and all, and that is awesomeness enough.

Stop Wishing, Start Doing.

We all have our wishes, our dreams, our goals. There is only one way to get there—taking that first step. Remind your child—especially on those tough days–that taking that first step is key. The rest will follow.

No Goal Was Ever Met Without A Little Sweat

Let's face it: our children are pretty spectacular. After all, they did spring from our loins and/or are graced by our presence and intelligence. However, that does not mean that their spectacularness will aid them in accomplishing their goals. As parents, one of the most important lessons we can teach our children is that despite their gifts and talents, it is their hard work and dedication that will dictate their success. We do our children a disservice when we brag about their talent and neglect focusing on their efforts.

"Believe you can and you are halfway there." Theodore Roosevelt

In middle and high school, our children are trying to figure out their place in the world—where they fit in. Doubts about their abilities and their struggles with confidence are front and center as they compare themselves with others, navigate new social circles, and explore new learning experiences. As parents, we can encourage confidence by reminding them of past successes and friendships. But remember, never minimize your child's feelings—they are real. With your support and reassurance and their attainment of new skills throughout their school career, they build up confidence and belief in their abilities.

Every Day is a Good Day to Workout

Okay, well some days are better than others to work out, quite honestly. So let us take the "workout" part away and focus on….every day is a good day. In my personal life, I have found appreciation for every day by counting blessings for the simple things: health, food on the table, clothes on my back, a sunny day, you know—all the stuff that brings us simple pleasures. Especially during these troubling times across the globe, we have so much to be thankful for: every day is a good day.

Now, let us put the "work out" part back in.

Yes, every day is a good day to workout. Teach your child the physical, mental/emotional, and social benefits of getting outside and walking, running, biking, gardening–whatever it is you enjoy. Physical activity releases endorphins that help people manage everyday stressors.

Last week I volunteered at a community fundraising event at a local middle school. Grandparents, parents, teachers, students, and siblings as young as three participated in the two-mile challenge. Enormous smiles were on the faces of the runners after their tremendous achievement, no matter how far they ran. Strangers engaged in animated conversation, congratulating each other on their accomplishment, forming a new community of friends. They learned life lessons about perseverance, supporting others, and gained an internal sense of accomplishment. Can you imagine the impact this school community event will have on these children down the road?

Yes, working out is a great thing—usually. However, finding inspiration that crosses over from the gym to career to raising children is an added bonus.

I wish you an awesome day of wishing, sweating, believing, and above all, goodness.

Quotes courtesy of Eric Warsaw, sweat-stc, LLC.

What's Next? Coping with a Teen's Disappointment

"Sometimes on the way to a dream you get lost and find another one.—Author unknown.

As many of you know, working out and running with friends or family lends itself to discussions one might not typically have. Try it with your child sometime when you have a serious topic to discuss. There are many reasons why discussion flows more easily during physical activity, and I have read some of the extensive research as to why this is. However, my own theory is that has to do with having a captive audience. (What are they going to do, run away from you? You will just catch up!) Or maybe it is a welcome distraction from the endless pounding of the feet on pavement during those particularly long runs.

It is the conversation, sharing, and bonding during physical exercise among friends and family that keep enthusiasts running week after week, year after year. Oh, yeah–and a few health benefits associated with running and exercising as well.

On a particularly lovely spring day as we pounded out the miles (okay, so we walked a lot), a story was relayed to me about a private conversation between a mother and her son. I found it very inspiring and knew I had to share this intimate moment with the world. (So, do not tell anyone, please.)

A young man, a sophomore in high school, tried out for the high school baseball team but did not make the roster. He is a great player but cuts needed to be made and he got the shaft. (Hearing this my heart ached for him, remembering the disappointments my own children experienced during their growing-up years.)

So the mom, devastated as she was, sought to comfort her son by suggesting they go out for coffee and just talk a while. What a thoughtful and loving gesture.

His response?

"Thanks, Mom. But can we go to the sports store? I want to try out for the track team this week and need new running shoes."

Wait…what?

No one threatened to call the coach to complain. No one whined about how unfair "it" is. No one sat around moping "woe is me." Instead, the young man stopped, looked around and said, "There is so much I can do in this world! What's next?!" What a refreshing perspective.

As parents, we *will* have to face disappointments alongside our children. It is tough for parents–when they hurt, we hurt even more. Yet based on this young man's response, it is clear his family understands the importance of moving forward when life throws a curve ball and has taught him well.

Yes, it is okay to feel disappointed, sad, frustrated, hurt–whatever your heart feels. We would be denying our authentic self if we ignored our unfavorable feelings. But after a good cry, use the dispiriting experience as a growth opportunity, and see what's next! Use your internal locus of control; look inside yourself to envision future possibilities. I firmly believe that when one door closes, a window opens–however *you* have to lift the window to see what is out there.

Put on your running shoes and get out there! The world is waiting for you and your family!

Challenges vs Disasters: Ten Ways to Help Your Child Prepare for the College Years

"They (college students) see every difficulty as a disaster, not a challenge. They've been made fragile by being overprotected, and this fragility is really harming them. It makes everything seem overwhelming."-Hara Estroff Marano, *Psychology Today*[5].

Intriguing quote, isn't it? I eagerly read the article in which this teaser is directing the reader. Found in the September/October 2015 *Psychology Today* issue, the article "Crisis U," brought home interesting and somewhat disturbing observances regarding current college students and their general mental health status. In the article, Marano states that over half of "college students report feeling overwhelming anxiety." Half. This is significant and demands our attention.

Because Marano addresses psychological issues current college students are facing, the parents that really need to understand and absorb this information are parents of students not in college—yet—to help break this trend of increasing anxiety.

The informative and well-researched article stressed me out. To alleviate my anxiety in a healthy manner, I thought I would share my thoughts. As parents, we have every right to be in our child's corner. In fact, we should! We can be terrific listeners, we can support their decisions, we can advise, we can encourage, we can suggest, and we can even offer to take them away for a fun weekend when they are feeling stressed. But what we should not do is coddle, baby, helicopter, and fill them with the idea that yes,

---

5   https://www.psychologytoday.com/articles/201509/crisis-u (2016) Crisis U

they are the best and yes, they deserve the best. Okay, okay. We *do* want the best for our children. It has been engrained in our brains to offer positive reinforcement to our children over every little accomplishment. (You ate all your green beans!? Awesome!) It seems, however, there is a balance when it comes to praising our spectacular kids.

What is best for our children is what they learn to give themselves: Self-efficacy. How we teach our kids to react to life situations as they grow and learn helps direct their energy and skills to cope with everyday stressors. Now, I am not talking about horrific, violent situations—that is beyond my scope. I am talking about the day-to-day issues of relationships, difficult classes, competition, job-hunting, and rejection. Stuff we all deal with. As Marano explores in her article, individuals can take these formidable situations and view them as debilitating stressors that knock them off their feet, or they can view the bumps-in-the-road as challenges that will enable them to grow as humans.

There are small steps parents can take to assist in the evolution of a self-reliant adult to have the intrinsic fortitude to tackle the inevitable life stressors awaiting our children.

1. At a school health conference I recently attended, teachers were encouraged to refrain from the comment "You are so smart!" when students do well. Rather, we were taught to focus on student's character and self-efficacy. For example, "I can tell you worked really hard on this" displaces the focus from being 'smart,' which labels a child, to work ethic and time invested in studying, which positively acknowledges their efforts. Parents you can do this, too. It takes a lot of practice to change our automatic response of over-the-top praise toward our child. After all, they really are so smart— just like we are!

2. Do not do your child's homework or other projects. Yes, they are dragging their feet. Yes, it would be soooo much easier if you shared the workload. But the child does not learn the consequence of turning work in late. They do not experience a sense of accomplishment that comes after each assignment. They learn to depend on others to do their work for them. They begin to feel they do not have the ability to succeed on their own. Besides, the teachers can often tell. You do not want to be that parent.

3. Allow your child to fail. This is a really hard one, I know. We want to cover for our children because we know they can do better, or someone else is to blame, or they had a bad day, or insert any number of excuses. But failure may inspire success the next time around as they learn from their mistakes, just as we did.

4. Model healthy stress-release activities such as running, reading, movies, socializing, and good old "talking it out" with a trusted person.

5. Help your child maintain focus on the "big picture." One failure, one break-up, one rejection does not mean their life is over, it merely means there is another class that needs to be taken, another person waiting to be loved, another job to be had—and often even better than before.

6. It is okay to express disappointment, hurt, rejection. We are human. But after a little time, encourage your child get back to living. It is a great big beautiful world out there, ready to entertain with new experiences and, well, more disappointment, too.

7. Refrain from continually voicing lofty expectations of your child. Ivy League school, pro ball player, medical school, valedictorian, collegiate superstar...whatever your fantasy is for your child, tone it down. Can you imagine how it must feel to have that kind of pressure on a kid? Yes, it is important to support and encourage them in their chosen areas of talent—it

is so much fun! However, your job is to help them realize that no matter where they go to school, how they place in an event, or if they get benched from a team, you embrace them for just being…them.

8. When your child is faced with particular stressors, share with them your own experiences. If you survived, they will, too.
9. Tell them you love them for who they are, warts and all, as we used to say.
10. Take it easy on yourself. There is no such thing as being a perfect parent any more than being a perfect child. We do our best with what we know.

By now you are wondering why I am even bothering to discuss stress when it has nothing to do with sex. But alas, if you read Marano's article, you will understand how increased stress can lead to an increased need for stress release. A need for increased stress release can lead to increased alcohol use/abuse. Excessive alcohol and drug use is a major factor in engaging in unsafe and unwanted sexual activity. The after effects of unwanted sexual activity is a huge issue on college campuses these days. And then of course, there is the STI issue. But I digress.

Had I been aware of the detriments of over-praising children, I could have adapted my parenting skills. However, in sending my girls far away to college and encouraging them to study abroad, the opportunity to hover like a helicopter was severed. Not that I would have if they were closer—I was pretty much ready to launch them, if you know what I mean. But, it was a great experience for all to send them on their way with a woeful wave and a tear in my eye, and the knowledge that I did the best I could with what I knew then. In fact, I believe my parting words for all three daughters were:

"You are now 18 and on your own. Your mistakes are your mistakes—I will not be there to fix them. However, I will always be here to love and support you. Your successes are your successes to enjoy and be proud of. Not mine. You got this. Now go conquer your world." Of course, I do take pride in their success. And I do give myself a little credit. After all, I did give them life.

It is the role of the parent, not the college, to teach their children how to bounce. College is a time to stop holding their hand for every little detail. It is wonderful when they call to share stories and ask for advice. I love giving advice (hence this book), but college is time to increase self-reliance. The years you invest in building their capability to resolve life's issues without feeling like every unfortunate event is a disaster will pay off. I get it— they are young adults who make decisions that cause you to roll your eyes, but they are getting there. We just need to get to get them to adulthood safely and with the appropriate life skills to allow them to be healthy and well-adjusted (well, semi-well-adjusted at least) adults. Just like your parents did for you.

Life is full of forks in the road. The adventure is exploring the paths ahead without fearing the unknown.

———————————

"I think they should talk about how to get out of situations that might force you to have sex." Female, 10th grade

"How to deal with relationship pressure." Male, 9th grade

"What is considered consent?" Female, 12th grade

"What is the sexual atmosphere like in college?" Female, 9th grade

PERSONAL SAFETY:

you can't hold their hand forever

Healthy Relationships:
Start the Conversation

February is Teen Dating Violence month. However, this is an issue that should spark conversation on a regular basis.

Take a look at these stats courtesy of *loveisrespect.org.*[1]

- Each year, one and a half million high schoolers are physically abused by their partner.
- Ten percent of high schoolers have been physically abused by their partner.
- One-third of teens have been abused by a partner, either physically, emotionally, sexually, or verbally.
- One-third of teens involved in an abusive relationship did not tell anyone about it.
- Twenty-five percent of high school females have been physically or sexually abused.

And here is one more statistic for you:

Over 80% of parents do not even realize teen dating violence is an issue.

It is wise to have the initial conversation about healthy relationships before your child begins dating, around late elementary school and into middle school. At that age, it may not be necessary to discuss teen dating violence. Rather, focus on exploring what a healthy relationship looks like.

---

1   http://www.loveisrespect.org/resources/dating-violence-statistics/ (2016) Dating Abuse Statistics

As your child grows older, they will become more aware of relationship violence merely by listening to music, watching TV and movies, or even in the halls of the school. You can use those experiences to build upon your ongoing conversations. Introducing dialogue about relationships at a young age will help keep the lines of communication open over the teenage years and beyond.

Follow these simple suggestions to initiate conversation:

1. Invite your son or daughter to coffee/tea/ice cream/dinner.
2. Forewarn them you have something you would like to talk to them about (but let them know they are not in trouble). It helps prepare them for an adult conversation.
3. As you joyfully dig into your ice cream sundae, explain to them that how much you love them. You will definitely get the eyeball roll, but that is okay—it means "I love you, too" in kid-speak.
4. Explain your desire for them to experience healthy friendships and romantic relationships now and in the future.
5. Let your child do the talking. You will learn more about your child by listening than by talking!
6. Be sure to ask open-ended questions. "Yes" and "no" questions will get you nowhere fast.

Now you actually have to converse. What should you talk about? How do you start? What do you say?Likely, the conversation will naturally progress. But if not, here are three important conversation starters and detailed talking points you can use.

Choose Your Own Conversation Adventure

1. "Tell me how you describe a healthy relationship."

Talking points:[2]

- What are your values? What is important to you? Do your friends and/or partner respect those values? How do you know? Do you respect their values? How do you show them? Do you share similar values?
- What are your goals and future plans? Do your friends and significant other support them? How do you know? Do you support their goals? How?
- Are you comfortable communicating to your friends and/or partner about your relationship when it comes to emotions and sex? How often do you have these conversations? Who usually approaches the subject? Do you feel respected when having these conversations? Do you respect their thoughts?
- Do you encourage each other to hang out with your own friends and family? How often do you call or text each other? How often do you hang out with people other than your significant other?
- How do you feel when you are with your partner? Happy, excited, valued? Uncomfortable, disappointed, confused?
- Do you feel safe with your partner? What makes you feel safe with them?
- Do you like your partner's friends?
- Is your partner quick to anger?
- Does your partner use drugs and/or alcohol and encourage you to do so, as well?

---

2   http://www.pamf.org/teen/abc/unhealthy/abuseforms.html (2013) Types of Abuse

2. "Tell me how you would recognize verbal abuse. Emotional abuse. Physical abuse. Sexual abuse."

Talking points

- General signs of abuse:[3]
  The person being abused may become withdrawn. Academically their grades may deteriorate. They may neglect their usual activities and relationships to spend all of their free time with their boyfriend/girlfriend. They may show physical signs of abuse such as bruising.
- Verbal abuse[4]:
  The abusive romantic partner may make insulting or cutting remarks towards their partner. They may say "just kidding!", but it is not funny. They may yell at their partner. They may become possessive or jealous by not allowing their partner to spend time with friends and family, telling them what to wear, and demanding to know their whereabouts at all times.
- Physical/sexual abuse:[5]
  The abusive romantic partner may hit, slap, or inflict other types of hurtful or inappropriate physical contact. They may force their partner to perform sex acts that they are not comfortable with or without consent. They may control what kind of birth control their partner is or is not permitted to use.

---

3   http://www.theredflagcampaign.org (2016) Healthy vs. Unhealthy Relationships
4   http://www.loveisrespect.org/is-this-abuse/types-of-abuse/#tab-id-2 (2016) Is This Abuse? Types of Abuse
5   http://www.pamf.org/teen/abc/unhealthy/abuseforms.html (2013) Types of Abuse

3. If you or someone you know is in an abusive relationship, what would you do?"

Talking points:

- Seek help from a trusted adult.
- School personnel, parents, and abuse hotlines can all offer help and advice.
- Break off the relationship, but follow safety guidelines.
- Do not be alone with your partner.
- Always let someone know where you are.
- Keep a phone with you at all times.
- Seek counseling. The effects of being abused can be far-reaching.

Tell your child that if they feel they are at risk of abusing someone they care about, seek professional help. There are excellent resources available. It's okay to ask for help—people care.

For more information about healthy relationships and teen dating violence, I recommend the following websites.

loveisrespect.org
breakthecycle.org
CDC.gov
datingabusestopshere.com
thehotline.org
vahealth.org
theredflagcampaign.org
teenshealth.org
pamf.org

Let's Talk: Consent and Sexual Assault

Currently, there is heated discussion circulating throughout social media and news media regarding the recent case of the young man convicted of three felonies related to sexual assault yet only sentenced to six months in prison[6]. Very few people are pleased with this verdict; many are outraged.

Disturbing to me is the lack of responsibility this man is taking for his actions. No, the alcohol did not digitally rape this young woman. No, frat culture did not assault this young woman. A clear and conscious choice to sexually gratify himself with an unconscious victim is evidenced by the hidden location of the assault–behind a garbage dumpster.

However, the most unsettling aspect of this, which keeps me up at night, is the support the rapist is receiving from other men– important men in his life–his dad and a representative of the law. It haunts me because it perpetuates the idea that rape is the victim's fault, not the offender's. The judge believes the young man did not commit a serious enough crime to ruin the rest of his life and does not feel he is a danger to society, despite the felony conviction. The dad believes his son's "twenty minutes of action" should not affect the rest of his life. Twenty minutes is a significant amount of time to participate in the assault of an unconscious woman without realizing, within the first few minutes, that what you are doing is very very wrong.

The message being sent is undeniably counter to what we are socially and humanly responsible for teaching all of our children: Respect others.

---

6   http://www.nytimes.com/2016/06/07/us/outrage-in-stanford-rape-case-over-dueling-statements-of-victim-and-attackers-father.html?_r=1 (2016) Light Sentence for Brock Turner in Stanford Rape Case Draws Outrage

The two heroic Swedish gentleman that came upon this horrific situation should be receiving our attention.

It is time to shift our focus from the asinine verdict that glorifies good 'ol boys to the young men who, without knowing if the perpetrator was armed, risked their own well-being to protect and assist a fellow human. This is the conversation we need to have with our children. Rather than having the felon's face on TV, I would prefer to gaze upon the two heroic Swedish men whose lives have also been forever altered by what they witnessed and experienced.

Let us show our youth the faces of upstanding men and women.

Let us show our youth what good character looks like.

Teaching young people respect for humankind needs to begin from the moment they have the ability to understand. Parents and other adults must model appropriate behavior towards others, demonstrate respect for others, and instruct their children in positive communication and relationship skills.

The brave survivor wrote a poignant letter to the perpetrator.[7] The moving, heart-wrenching letter she wrote should be required reading for all high school students. Reading the powerful, fervent words of this survivor will have an impact unequaled to anything taught in a textbook. That letter, so compelling and beautifully written, also serves as a mental refuge for the millions of other women who have been and are continually violated.

Sexual abuse of women is rampant. According to the *National Sexual Violence Resource Center*, "one in five women and one in 16 men are sexually assaulted in college:" 90% of these assaults are not

---

7   https://www.buzzfeed.com/katiejmbaker/heres-the-powerful-letter-the-stanford-victim-read-to-her-ra?utm_term=.oe0Dw6PN4#.av5qn3odB (2016) Here Is The Powerful Letter The Stanford Victim Read Aloud To Her Attacker

reported. Additionally, approximately 63% of men who admitted to committing these crimes also stated they had done so on more than one occasion.[8] Campus rape is nothing new; but the conversation, tolerance, and awareness of the issue is exploding.

Teaching our children to be "upstanders," not merely bystanders, is crucial. An upstander is someone who proactively supports those who may be targeted by bullies and perpetrators. These individuals focus on being a positive influence in their community. An upstander is someone who, when observing an inebriated young woman walking out of a party alone or with a person with questionable intentions, intervenes to ensure this individual arrives home safely.

- Teach our young people to help one another in times of need.
- Be mindful of the messages our young people are inundated with daily. Use media informed stories as opportunities to spark open and honest conversation.
- Focus on positive examples of humanity in your own family, community, and the world. There are so many amazing, caring people.
- Encourage your children to be upstanders.
- Lead by example.

The ripples of change being left by this outrageous oceanic disturbance has allowed a chorus of voices to be heard over the roaring wave of complacency when it comes to sexual violence. Let your child hear your wise voice.

---

8 http://www.nsvrc.org/sites/default/files/publications_nsvrc_factsheet_media-packet_statistics-about-sexual-violence_0.pdf (2015) Statistics about Sexual Violence

100 Percent of the Time:
Campus Sexual Assault

After a particularly lovely Sunday Funday enjoying one of the last weekends of summer, a close friends and her daughter decided to linger a little longer. (Girl Scout cookies anyone?)

Her daughter will be leaving the nest soon to attend college–very far away. With every parent facing the prospect of their child hurdling this milestone, there are worries. We don't know exactly what their adventures, challenges, or even their successes will be. They won't come home at the end of the day to share their concerns and issues with you. You won't be able to look them in the eyes and get a sense of their mood. It's a difficult transition–for adults as well as youth.

Young adults moving on to college, or even moving to their own space, will be faced with issues beyond "are my socks clean?" The issues may be life-changing–for better or worse. Not only will they have to worry about laundry, but they are responsible for getting themselves to class, and they will take on financial responsibilities. Socially, they will meet new people with different life experiences and perspectives. They will develop life-long relationships, begin attending parties not supervised by adults, and start dating people that parents have not met. These young adults will have to rely on their own common sense and judgement when it comes to making decisions. But as we all know, "you can't be old and wise without being young and crazy." At least that is what I have heard.

As responsible adults, we have done what we can to make them accountable for their actions. But then again, so did our parents when we were that age. And we all know how well *that* turned out, right? Admit it...you made some, um, "interesting" choices back in the day, too.

The best thing is to arm them with information, advice, support, and love...because the issues facing our young adults are not always as mundane as clean socks.

So, when my friend asked me to talk to her daughter about campus rape, I looked at this beautiful and sweet young woman and thought to myself: "Going back in time, when my own daughters were leaving for their new life adventures, what did I tell them? What would I tell them now–after all the research and understanding I have of the topic?"

It is an incredibly serious and scary topic, but we do not want to send them into the world untrusting and afraid of what lies ahead. However, knowledge is power, and the more they understand, the safer they might be. At least that is how I feel.

When my oldest left for college 9 years ago, then the next one 3 years later, then the "baby" 3 years after that, my advice was the same for each. "Always go out with friends, never alone; always return home with the same friends, never leave anyone behind. Ever." "Never set your glass down and walk away." "Never let someone serve you a drink. You don't know what they put into that cup while you weren't looking." Pretty succinct advice–short, practical, and easy to follow. In fact, I would still offer that advice. 100%. I would offer this to both males and females–no one is excluded from being victimized.

However, the statistics are alarming. The stories are disturbing. And the aftermath of a rape/sexual assault is, well, you wouldn't believe it if I told you. There have been numerous reports over the years about campus rape: Who are the victims? Who are the perpetrators? Where does this happen? What factors are involved? Who is at fault? And what kind of help is available for the victims?

100% of the time it is *not* the victim's fault.

100% of the time, the person who made the decision to assault is at fault. Period.

Historically, victims of sexual assault not only have to deal with the assault itself, but they also have to deal with a system that prefers to push the issue under the rug.

Recently, there has been a push for colleges to make public the specific incidences of sexual assault reported on-and off-campus to encourage accountability. This push has inspired several mainstream magazines to report about the rape culture on campus, and what is–and is not–being done to enable students to learn and live in the safest environment possible. TIME magazine published a piece by Eliza Gray on May 26, 2014 about campus rape called *"The Crisis in Higher Education."*[9] Also, Rolling Stone magazine published an article called *"Confronting Campus Rape"* by Nina Burleigh on June 19, 2014.[10] Both are excellent articles addressing campus sexual assault.

For decades, Joe Biden has been a fervent supporter of stricter regulations when it comes to campus sexual assault. Recently he joined forces with the Obama administration to crack down on universities who downplay or ignore reports of assault and rape.[11] They have even begun a program called *It's On Us* which encourages college students to take a pledge to be proactive and support efforts to decrease campus sexual violence. [12] (ItsOnUs.org)

---

9   https://blog.ecu.edu/sites/dailyclips/blog/2014/05/27/the-sexual-assault-crisis-on-american-campuses-time-magazine (2014) The Sexual Assault Crisis on American Campuses | Time Magazine

10 http://www.rollingstone.com/politics/news/confronting-campus-rape-20140604 (2014) Confronting Campus Rape

11 https://www.washingtonpost.com/politics/biden-and-obama-rewrite-the-rulebook-on-college-sexual-assaults/2016/07/03/0773302e-3654-11e6-a254-2b336e293a3c_story.html (2016)
    Biden and Obama rewrite the rulebook on college sexual assaults

12 https://www.whitehouse.gov/blog/2014/09/19/president-obama-launches-its-us-campaign-end-sexual-assault-campus (2014) President Obama Launches the "It's On Us" Campaign to End Sexual Assault on Campus

So what do we know? A study was commissioned by the Department of Justice to find out exactly what is happening on college campuses. The following statistics are from that study: *The Campus Sexual Assault Study.*[13]

- 19% of women will be the victim of sexual assault or attempted sexual assault during college.
- That's almost 20%. One in five.
  Of the study participants who had been sexually assaulted or an attempt was made:
- 89% had been drinking.
- 61% of sexual assaults happened off-campus.
- 58% of sexual assaults had been at a party.
- 28% were assaulted by a fraternity member.
- 2.3% of the time the victim suspected or was certain they were unknowingly drugged.
- 85-90% know their assailant.
- 64% to 96% of all rapes are not reported to authorities.
- 6.4% of men commit sexual assaults. Half are repeat offenders–with an average of 6 rapes each.

Interesting, isn't it, that it's the same guys repeating the crime. As reported in Gray's article, it was found that the guys who are victimizing the coeds actually have a bit of a plan. They look for certain women to sexually assault. They are often attractive freshman and sophomores who are finally out from under an adult's watchful eye. They may binge-drink and don't yet know their safe alcohol limit. They are easy targets in which to encourage intoxication. Alcohol may make the victim unable to make a safe decision, or the perpetrator may take advantage of the young woman if she has passed out. The rapist understands that if alcohol is involved, the odds of being convicted of rape are low–after all, she was drunk.

Yes, alcohol is the weapon.

13 https://www.ncjrs.gov/pdffiles1/nij/grants/221153.pdf (2007) The Campus Sexual Assault (CSA) Study

According to *Northwestern University's Women's Center*[14]:

- A person who is asleep or mentally or physically incapacitated, either through the effect of drugs or alcohol or for any other reason, is not capable of giving valid consent.
- The use of alcohol or drugs may seriously interfere with the participants' judgment about whether consent has been sought and given.

100% of the time it is *not* the victim's fault.

What will you tell your son or daughter when they leave for college? Explain personal safety, but also discuss ways to help discourage and prevent campus sexual assault. It's on us.

---

14 http://www.northwestern.edu/womenscenter (2016) Defining Sexual Assault

Sexual Harassment. It's All Business

It is not often I read the business section of the newspaper on Sunday mornings. Rather, I tend to gravitate towards the **Travel and Lifestyle** sections. I rarely miss a column by Heidi Stevens. The weekly column *I Just Work Here* is written by Rex W. Huppke. I admit, I rarely read it. Okay, I have never read it. After all, it is in the Chicago Tribune business section! Big yawn. However, a headline on the front of the business section grabbed my attention:

*Male Allies Should Call Out Harassers**

---

*   http://www.chicagotribune.com/business/careers/ijustworkhere/ct-huppke-work-advice-sexual-harassment-0911-biz-20160908-column.html

Hey, this is something I write about as a health educator. In the business section?! Heidi would have to wait.

In the article, Huppke discusses the perturbing events highlighted by recent newscasts about the Fox News sexual harassment case. Using that situation as a platform, he delves into typical office shenanigans that happen on a daily basis in businesses everywhere and questions: "Where are the men in this?"

He argues it is time that men, not just women, step up and shut down any comments, innuendos, and inappropriate sexual transgressions that are offensive and unprofessional towards women.

As educators and parents, it is imperative we teach our boys and young men the importance of respecting women. Huppke is encouraging educating and mentoring as well, but in all places, the business section of a newspaper!?

Hmmm. Now that I think about it, what better place? In a business environment, young professionals are learning the ropes from seasoned pros. Perhaps what is learned in the workplace is carried through to their social life. We need men of integrity to lead by standing up for what is appropriate, professional, and just plain considerate.

I love the challenge that Huppke is presenting to professional men. Heck, all men. Huppke states: "*A real man has the guts to stand up to behavior that harms others. And in the case of sexual harassment, in all its forms, I think we need more real men to lend a hand.*"

Well said.

Avoiding Unsafe Situations

It is early Saturday morning. I usually head out for a long run. Today, however, an injury is keeping me from hitting the tranquil trail. Not to mention the nonstop rain. I pour myself a cup of coffee to fire the cylinders in my brain and settle in to watch the national news.

The first news segment to catch my attention announced that a young man at an East Coast prep school had been found guilty of statutory rape, not felony sexual assault charges., as most people at expected.

I am not a lawyer or judge, nor was I a member of the jury. The laws are clear, but the situation is murky. He said, she said. What is true? What is real? It seems this scenario is being played out with more frequency, especially among athletes. It is not my job to convict. However, I would like to take this opportunity to educate parents on the importance of conversation with your child to help prevent these situations from traumatizing your family.

"Stranger Danger" is a concept parents grapple with almost the moment our precious being arrives into our world. The fears perpetuated by unsavory news stories suddenly hit home. Certainly we do not want our children to be unfriendly to strangers–after all, most people are kind and wonderful. However, what if they are not? What if they are creepy? Who knew Jared the Subway guy would turn out to have, shall we say…"issues"? *Jared*?!

When children are small, we have basic conversations with them regarding safety.

- We explain to children about good touch, bad touch.

- We devise special "code words" that only other trusted adults will know just in case we are unable to pick them up from an activity. These are "safe people" our children can trust.
- We teach children to keep their distance from people they do not know, yet smiles and greetings are still okay.
- We explain that only adults should assist other adults. That lost puppy Mr. Danger needs help locating is not their responsibility.
- Finally, one of the most important lessons we can begin teaching our young kids is to follow their gut. If something does not feel right, then it probably is not. It is a tough concept for adults, much less kids. However, it is an important aspect of learning self-reliance.

When looking at the above list of safety concepts we instill in our children, there is a common thread:

If a situation does not feel or look safe, avoid it.

As our kids grow older, they have more freedom, gain more independence, and meet new people of all ages. They begin to date—first in group situations, then as couples. Before you know it, they are off to college. No longer are you with them on a daily basis, assessing their mental/emotional state as parents tend to do. No longer are you able to look them in the eye to see if something is troubling them. No longer are you able to meet the men and women in their lives that can significantly impact their world. You hope what you taught them about being safe and responsible as they were growing will surface when the situation warrants. In other words, you hope that they remember the simple idea that:

If a situation does not feel or look safe, avoid it.

Because the statutory rape of the student happened within the confines of an educational institution, it is imperative that learning institutions take notice and address these tough issues with their students. Instituting comprehensive sexuality heath education (CSE) beginning with the youngest of students is a conversation that is completely overdue. Yes, that is correct. Even in kindergarten. Learning about respect for self and others, healthy relationships, and how to navigate around unsafe and uncomfortable situations is a major component of this type of education.

As students move into higher grade levels, they are faced with very real situations that require considerate and thoughtful responses. These assertive responses should be predetermined and practiced before the situation hits them head-on. Starting the conversations in kindergarten and building upon that knowledge rather than waiting until high school when discussion is 'too little, too late' is a change that is overdue.

CSE curriculum offers guidance and reflection on students' future goals and how to reach those aspirations. It focuses on decision-making, respect for others, and personal safety. It offers opportunity for discussion among students of all identities and orientations to enable understanding and mutual respect.

So, what can parents do to help our young people navigate unhealthy situations?

- Start the conversation with our children at a young age about appropriate touch, gut-instinct, goals, and respecting others.
- Explain to our young people that is it okay to be "rude" and walk away when a situation doesn't "feel" right, or if someone is making unwelcome advances.

- Keep the conversation alive with your child. Media-driven discussion makes it easy. My daughter and I have had several conversations about the many high profile rape charges dotting news reports lately.
- Ask open-ended questions that allow your child to give thoughtful responses about safe and unsafe situations.
- Encourage schools to adopt CSE curriculum so students benefit from co-ed discussion and diverse perspective.
- Talk about consent.

As parents, we spend much of our conversation educating, or rather sermonizing, our kids–"don't do this, don't do that." Lecturing kids is not the most effective approach. Granted, your children do need to know how you feel; your family rules and expectations convey your value system and sets limits on behavior. That is a good thing. However intrinsic desire to make good choices, not merely rules and regulations, is the most effective means to keep children as safe as possible when making choices to drink, drug, engage in sex, or any other decisions they may be faced with.

Yes, I know. Merely adopting the mantra of "if a situation does not look or feel safe, avoid it" will not keep our children from facing situations that are compromising. If only life were that simple. However, by instilling the idea that we can make decisions that are wise and responsible, we give our children just one more life skill they can intrinsically rely on as they emerge into the adult world.

Let's Talk: Sexually Assaulted Males

Society tends to place a greater eye on female victimization when it comes to rape and sexual assault. I get that. It's pretty scary to think about the physical strength of a male vs. the strength of a female and the odds of defending herself. There's a bit of testosterone involved. However females are not the only victims of rape, and we are doing society a disservice by neglecting this important reality.

As we know, instances of sexual assault and rape are markedly underreported for many reasons. According to the *National Institute of Justice*, these are some of the more common reasons that men and women do not report sexual abuse[15]:

- shame
- embarrassment
- lack of support by authorities
- humiliation
- distrust of legal system
- guilt
- privacy
- fear of retribution
- afraid of what others will think.

Consider this: what if a male is physically or psychologically forced into having sex, either by a man or woman? There is an untruth that all guys "want it," therefore males cannot be raped. Another fallacy is if a man is raped, he must identify as gay. Imagine how difficult it would be to report the assault when the societal assumptions about male sexuality are so skewed.

---

15 http://www.nij.gov/topics/crime/rape-sexual-violence/Pages/welcome.aspx
(2016) Rape and Sexual Violence

We are all familiar with the media accounts of men in power who have sexually assaulted and abused young boys and men. Religious leaders, teachers, a university football coach…all using their authority to coerce males for their sexual pleasure and/or to demonstrate their dominance. But women can do the same.

According to Sally Strosahl, M.A., LCPC, male sexual assault is more common than we realize, and the psychological effects on the male victim can be devastating, just as it is for other sexes (female and intersex*). She relayed the following story about a high school male with whom she had the privilege to counsel.

---

*   Intersex: A person is born with ambiguous male and female anatomy–external as well as internal. Sometimes it is obvious at birth, other times it isn't noticed until puberty, and sometimes a person never knows! There are several medical conditions associated with being intersex, including Turner Syndrome and Klinefelter Syndrome. This has nothing to do with sexual orientation.

"Mike (not his real name) began to close himself off from friends and family. He often retreated to his bedroom after dinner rather than engage with the family as he usually had in the past. His appetite decreased as well and he began to lose weight.

Mike, who is typically upbeat and easygoing, suddenly became surly and easily irritated. As his personality continued down a negative path, his parents recognized this as an indicator of depression and sought out my therapeutic services.

After the first couple of sessions, he began sharing personal details about his relationship with his girlfriend. She was a bit older; a senior in contrast to his sophomore status.

Mike wasn't quite ready for a sexual relationship, though he did enjoy time spent together. However, his girlfriend had different ideas and wanted to engage in sexual activity with this young man. Using psychological coercion, she forced him into a physically intimate relationship despite his preference to wait until he was ready.

Using threats such as, "If you don't have sex with me, I'll tell everyone you have a small penis," or derogatory statements such as, "I don't know why I bother going out with you. You have no idea how lucky you are to have me." She was psychologically abusive by taking advantage of his vulnerability. Mentally beating Mike down, his "girlfriend" coerced him to have sex–otherwise known as rape. However, this young woman soon grew bored with him and broke it off, possibly going on to her next sexual conquest.

After several sessions of therapeutic work, he slowly came to understand that he was a victim of rape, sexual abuse, and emotional abuse. Eventually he met a new girl–his age–and has a healthy relationship thanks to the hard work this young man went through with counseling and with the support of his parents.

I want to emphasize that as awful as rape and sexual assault is for a victim, not getting the appropriate psychological help to recover can make the situation infinitely worse. I encourage all victims of abuse–sexual or other–to seek help. It is not your fault–no matter if you are male or female. Get help."

Sexual assault of men is real. Because of the social stigma attached to it, reporting is incredibly low. According to the *Sexual Assault Response Services of Southern Maine*, 61% of all rapes are not reported.[16] Male-only statistics are harder to come by because of the lack of reporting. Being aware that this actually occurs is the first step in advocating for these individuals. According to *The*

---

16 http://www.sarsonline.org Sexual Assault and Rape Statistics, Laws, and Reports

Campus Sexual Assault Study researched by *RTI International,* since entering a college campus, 6.1% of men experienced an attempted or completed sexual assault.

I happened upon this interesting article *"When Men Are Raped"* by Hanna Rosin.[17] For further investigation about men who are sexually assaulted, I recommend this article.

Would you like more information or support? Please go to these links. You are *not* alone.

RAINN
PANDORA'S PROJECT
1 IN 6
MEN CAN STOP RAPE
BAND BACK TOGETHER
Universities also offer support and counseling.

---

17 http://www.slate.com/articles/double_x/doublex/2014/04/male_rape_in_
america_a_new_study_reveals_that_men_are_sexually_assaulted.html (2014)
When Men Are Raped

Sex Trafficking: Talking to Your Child about Internet and Community Safety

Several years ago, I had an unforgettable experience. To this day it troubles me.

I arrived from a vacation and proceeded to collect my car from a privately owned parking lot just outside the airport. As I waited in the tired soulless lobby for my keys, I observed a young girl, maybe about age 12 or so, and a much younger girl with her. They both looked exhausted, staring out the big picture window at the grey scene before them.

One of the girls wore fashionable grown-up platform shoes and a revealing dress designed for a mature woman. (I do not recall what the younger girl wore.) None of this made sense to me: Where are the parents? Why is this child dressed like an adult? Who are they waiting for? Why are they so exhausted? Why here?

Where are their innocent childlike smiles?

That scene has haunted me for several years now. My instinct told me something was amiss. But what exactly? I was able to logically explain away each concern: Kids like to play dress-up, parents left to grab their car, tired from traveling.

Mom-instinct told me otherwise.

Recently, I attended a seminar for school health educators and nurses in which the topic of sex/human trafficking was presented. As the facts and stats were presented, the scene in the airport carpark came rushing back to me.

What had I witnessed? Something completely innocent? Something disturbing? I will never know; yet I do know what to do next time.

Following the seminar, I contacted one of the presenters. We spoke about this important topic. Because of the nature of her work, she requested anonymity, which I respect. She offered some interesting and helpful information I feel compelled to share.

It is not unusual for traffickers to target individuals who are vulnerable due to their life situations.

- Young people who feel lonely or dismissed by parents may respond to a person who spends time with them and "respects" them.
- People who may be going through difficult personal situations such as a parental divorce and the stressors associated with that life change and do not have appropriate support may be vulnerable.
- Homeless young people who deal with a myriad of issues that traffickers can hone in on are easy prey.
- Girls who may have low self-esteem and are trying to find their place in the world can fall victim.
- Individuals who identify as LGBTQ could be more vulnerable. According to the *Polaris Project*, the LGBT population is *five times* more likely to be targeted by traffickers. Why? Think about the struggle this population goes through to just have the same basic rights as straight citizens. Feeling marginalized, unwanted, isolated, and alone, this population is particularly vulnerable to these predators who swoop in to offer acceptance and community.

Predators look for targets in a variety of hang outs:

- social media such as Facebook
- through friends
- as a result of contacts made with drug users
- malls
- amusement parks
- even gas stations

How does one fall victim to sex traffickers?

- physically forced
- victims of fraud—they are promised something, like clothes, drugs, or even love, yet they do not receive what it is they truly want
- threatened until they comply

Talking with your children about safety, both internet and within the community, is imperative.

- Help them understand why you want to have the conversation. You want them to be aware, not frightened.
- Approach the topic with logic and love, not anger or anxiety.
- Stress how much you care for your child, are proud to be their mother or father, and just want them safe.
- Avoid blaming.
- Remind them that if they find themselves in scary situations, you are always there for them no matter what.
- Tell them it is okay to report any uncomfortable situation.
- Remind them to follow the little voice that says "bad idea". It may not be very loud, but listen to the whisper.
- Ask open-ended questions. According to *netsmartz.org*, conversations can be lead with questions such as:
  - "What would you do if…"

- "Has anyone ever…"
- "Why and how might someone try to gain your trust?"
- Teach online safety basics:
- Never give out personal information.
- Never share photos in private messages.
- Anything posted on social media is permanent.
- No sexting.
- Never accept a "friend" request from someone they do not know.

Be proactive parents.

- Use parental controls to keep their viewing habits in check;
- Check their browsing history. If they are on *Back Page* or *Craig's List*, a little red flag should go up. Those sites may be looking for young people to traffic.
- Keep the conversations flowing.
- Set up family guidelines for internet use.
- Show interest in your child's viewing habits.
- Report suspicious activity to the authorities without hesitation.

What is the best protection for your child to avoid falling victim to predators?

BE. THERE. FOR. THEM. Be present and engaged. No, you can't be there all the time, of course. However, dismissing a child with $20 and a routine "go make yourself scarce" attitude could be asking for trouble. Rather, use that money for a fun excursion with your child on a regular basis. Quarterly, monthly, weekly… doesn't matter as long as you use that time to connect. The bond you form during your dedicated time together will spill over into daily life as you navigate routine challenges. Not always, but enough. Your child wants your time.

If your family is struggling with personal issues such as divorce or homelessness, reach out for social service help or counseling. Talk to your child's school personnel. You'll be amazed how effective it is to have trusted adults, even just one, within your child's school community.

In other words, all kids have stressors. They need the adults in their lives to step up. If they don't, they will find someone who will.

Sex trafficking is incredibly complex and multifaceted. I cannot even begin to pretend I am an expert. Yet my experience at the airport car park offered me the realization that anyone of us may unexpectedly be faced with sex trafficking.

So, what does a concerned citizen do if they find themselves in a situation similar to my experience at the airport car lot?

9-1-1.

Local police agencies have been trained on what to look for. It was suggested by the anonymous law enforcement person I interviewed to simply state your observations, your location, and that you may be totally wrong but just wanted to be on the safe side. You can also call 1-800-843-5678 or go to www.cybertipline.org. However, in those moments when you are faced with a split-second decision circumstance just call 9-1-1.

For more information, these following sites are outstanding and comprehensive for parents, educators, law enforcement personnel, and even teens. These sites are under the umbrella of the *National Center for Missing and Exploited Children (NCMEC)*.
netsmartz.org (*Great for families, educators, and law enforcement professionals.*)

Polaris Project.org (Information about legal issues and trafficking.)
National Human Trafficking Resource Center (NHTRC.org) (Great for educators.)
Missing Kids.org (The homepage for NCMEC.)

Bullying: Let's Change the Channel

Bullying...something we hope our children don't experience–or instigate. Even if they do not experience bullying directly, 56% of students have been bystanders and witnessed bullying in the school setting.[18] Odds are, your child or their friends will indeed be affected by bullying. With the school year just beginning, now is a good time to be armed with strategies to assist the young person in your life when faced with this issue.

Bullying occurs when a person or persons repeatedly harms or threatens another person either verbally, physically, emotionally, or socially. This can be done directly (hitting, teasing, threatening) or indirectly (starting rumors, leaving someone out on purpose).

I won't spend our time going through all the effects bullying can have on a person. We all know it can increase anxiety and depression. It can decrease self-esteem. The child may not want to attend school, and is likely to skip PE. (Guess where a lot of bullying takes place while in school?) The effects can last a lifetime.

So what do we do?

1. Labeling people as "bullies" and "victims" is not a great idea. Labeling a person implies this is who they are and who they will always be, and we don't want these young people to carry that label into adulthood–we want them to grow into confident, compassionate humans.
2. Model empathy and kindness. Avoid disparaging remarks about others, especially those who identify as a minority within your community; someone who is "different" than you as far as race, religion, culture, sexual orientation, or economic status. Typically, these individuals become the targets of those that bully.

---

18 http://familyplacebeproject.org Bullying The Statistics

3. Understand the social messages that inundate our society. Reality shows frequently model belittling between individuals. I just don't find that entertaining; in fact, I find it hurtful and painful to watch. The message we send to people, regardless of age, is that by insulting others, people can appear more confident and powerful. The truth is, the person doing the belittling is probably dealing with their own feelings of insecurity, or have experienced bullying themselves. They haven't learned social skills that enable them to communicate effectively without using hurtful messages. We also hear controlling messages in music, and experience less-than-friendly rivalry with certain sporting events, such as wrestling.[19] Start a conversation with your young person about these messages.

4. Focus on positive behavior. When you see a young person being kind to someone, remark on it. However, focus on what the child did and what the outcome was, not how you feel about what the child just did. For example, "I noticed you helped Richard get away from Tom when he was teased. He looked relieved."[20] That can inspire the child to be kind because it makes *him* feel good about his actions, not because it makes *you* feel good or proud.

5. Talk about bullying. Explain bullying is never okay, and that it is important to tell an adult if it happens to them or a peer. According to stopbullying.gov, give them strategies such as telling the person doing the bullying to stop–but do not confront–then walk away.[21] Or disarm him with humor, then walk away. Or just walk away. (Get the pattern here?) An adult should be informed–or tell friends–so s/he won't feel so alone. Walk in groups of friends or stick by adults, since it isn't as likely to happen if there are adults around.

---

19 http://www.bullyingstatistics.org Facts About School Bullies and Bullying Behaviors
20 http://www.maine.gov/education/guidelines.htm (2006) Guidelines for Effective Discussions About Bullying
21 https://www.stopbullying.gov (2016) Support The Kids Involved

6. Look for tell-tale signs that your child may be having problems. Classic signs include increased anxiety and depression, falling grades, or feeling "too sick" to go to school. Locker room bullying before and after PE class, as well as during class, is common. Playground bullying as well as during intramural sports are other typical bully opportunities. If your child or student refuses to dress for PE, attend PE class, or decides they no longer want to play on a team or go out for recess, red flags should be going up.[22]

7. Be there for your child. Ask them open-ended questions about their day. Ask who they hang with, eat with, talk to. Show them you are there for them.

8. Many kids are bystanders, that is, they witness the bullying, but don't know what to do. I totally get that. There is a fear of becoming a victim themselves. But when that happens, the person who bullies has an audience, which they like, and they also take the silence as approval and encouragement. So let's have them try these strategies offered by Stan Davis of StopBullyingNow.org and StopBullying.gov.

   • Help the person being bullied escape by telling him he is needed elsewhere and then walking out with him.
   • If someone is sharing a rumor, change the subject.
   • Do not spread rumors, and tell friends to not share rumors as well.
   • Spend time with or become friends with the person who is being bullied so they don't feel alone.
   • Tell a trusted adult.

9. One other interesting tidbit to keep in mind. According to Bullying Prevention of the State of Maine and Stan Davis, encouraging a student to talk with the person who bullied

---

22 Roman, C., & Taylor, C. (2013). A Multilevel Assessment of School Climate, Bullying Victimization, and Physical Activity. Journal of School Health, 83(6), 400-407.

them to explain how they feel is a big no-no. By telling that person they feel hurt, sad, mad...whatever...s/he has gained power over their target that they were seeking–their bullying worked! It won't stop the behavior, in fact it may make the problem worse. Remember, this isn't a squabble between two friends.

This goes beyond "it's not nice" to bully. How can we change our social constructs so that good deeds demand more of our focus than negativity? TV, music, movies, sports, news, daily conversation... be aware of the subtle messages our youth are receiving. We can't change what is on TV, but we can change the channel.

If Fun is the Goal, is Drinking the Objective?: Making Wise Decisions

"The perfect beer for removing 'no' from your vocabulary for the night."

The marketing experts behind a prominent beer maker made the mistake of creating this ignorant advice and printing it on some of their bottles. Their campaign #UpForWhatever is meant to inspire people to venture outside their box and have new experiences. Okay. I get that. In fact, I encourage people to try new things. What concerns me, however, is encouraging people who have been drinking to do #whatever they want; alcohol inspires people to ignore logic.

We already have a problem with poor decision-making skills when it comes to alcohol use. According to one study, alcohol is involved in half of all violent crimes, including sexual assault.[23] Thirty people die every day from car accidents in which alcohol is involved.[24] In 2012, there were 140 boating accident deaths related to alcohol consumption.[25]

Binge-drinking is considered risky behavior when it comes to sexual decision-making.[26] Unprotected sex and/or having more than one partner increases a person's odds of contracting an STI or becoming

---

23 http://pubs.niaaa.nih.gov/publications/arh25-1/43-51.htmAlcohol and Sexual Assault Antonia Abbey, Ph.D., Tina Zawacki, M.A., Philip O. Buck, M.A., A. Monique Clinton, M.A., and Pam McAuslan, Ph.D

24 http://www.cdc.gov/Motorvehiclesafety/impaired_driving/impaired-drv_factsheet.html (2016) Impaired Driving: Get the Facts

25 http://uscgboating.org/library/accident-statistics/834.PDF (2012) 2012 Recreational Boating Statistics

26 http://www.cdc.gov/alcohol/fact-sheets/alcohol-use.htm (2016) Fact Sheets: Alcohol Use and Your Health

pregnant. In fact, a British study showed that at one clinic, patients diagnosed with an STI consumed 40% more alcohol each week than their STI-free counterparts.[27]

Encouraging individuals to say "yes" to any opportunity that presents itself while drinking is irresponsible at best. Marrying this misleading recommendation with the party-atmosphere ads that typically surround alcohol advertising promote the idea that, if fun is the goal, then drinking is the objective.

Conversation with your child about responsible drinking should begin at a young age. It is sort of like sex:

You know it will happen…
You don't know when…
But when it does, you want them to be safe.

Encourage your kids to get out there and explore the world. Have them step outside their comfort zone and try new experiences. But before they do, hand them a frosty glass of…lemonade.

Adolescents do not need a beer ad to encourage them to spread their wings…they have you!

———————————

27 http://www.womens-health.co.uk/alcohol-and-stds.html (2016) Alcohol and STDs

Good Vibrations: Talking to Your Kids About Drinking, Hydration, and Music Fests

As former teenagers, we get it. As parents, we don't.

Summer, in all its glory, tempts even the "best" kids with sizzling summer romance, impromptu parentless parties, and yes, even cheap alcohol (Boone's Farm anyone?) to fuel fleeting summer excitement. Ah, yes. The cool kids partying in the summer. That was never me. But I'm cool now. Totally cool. I really am. Trust me.

Music enhances summer exhilaration as teens converge in the twilight hours to share a few stolen beers and (hopefully) innocent kisses. Remember "Summer Nights" from Grease? "All Summer Long" by Kid Rock? "Summer in the City" by Lovin' Spoonful? "Summertime" by Janis? "Summer of '69" by Bryan Adams? "In the Summertime" by Mungo Jerry? Pretty much anything by the Beach Boys? Ah, the memories.

Okay, I'm dating myself, but just tell me these immortalized songs don't bring back a tingle of wistful memories lost in the recesses of your mind. You can thank me later. Of course, now we are responsible parents who have buried those sweet summer sensations and replaced them with endless swim lessons, park district programs, visits to the pool, and reading incentive programs (my personal favorite).

Our teens eagerly head out for the evening as we shout, "Don't forget curfew!!" "Make good choices!" "I'll be waiting up for you to smell your breath!" Frankly, I think they tune out the minute we open our mouths, but hey, at least we said our piece .

Unfortunately, it is not all fun and games. Recently, a local news station presented an engaging report about music festivals, alcohol poisoning, and young people. I hesitate to say teens, because quite frankly, it can happen to anyone. However, teens seem to have an especially difficult time reading the "STOP!" cues from their immature brains.

In Chicago, Lollapalooza is one of the biggest events of the year. It is a blast–one of my favorite life memories. Unfortunately, I believe I've "aged out" of the event. Lolla is scorching hot. The days are long. The bands are exciting. It is crowded beyond crowded. There are several water stations, but there are long lines. Lots of lines, for everything. In other words, even if alcohol isn't involved, it is a risky event merely by being in the hot, unforgiving sun. Yes, people must have wristbands to obtain alcohol, but with tens of thousands of people present, we know how well that works.

Discuss ways in which your child can stay safe. Here's a cheat sheet to assist you with tips.

- Don't drink alcohol.
- Hydrate after each alcoholic drink they (don't) drink.
- Get out of the heat as often as possible.
- Be sure to have emergency contact info on the wristbands and on their phone, as suggested by the report.
- Chaperone your child, or at least have someone in the general area of the event.
- Call or text your child frequently. Okay, just occasionally or they may stop responding.
- Don't freak out if they don't answer the phone right away–it is really, really loud at concerts, remember?
- Explain the consequences related to bad decision-making.
- Discuss safety measures if a friend over-imbibes.[28] (Hydrate,

---

28

get out of the sun, call 911 or bring them to a first aid tent. Turn them to their side to prevent aspiration of vomit. Keep in mind alcohol is a depressant. That means if a person drinks too much, it can depress their body systems, including the respiratory system. If their respiratory system is depressed, it won't work. That is a big deal. We need oxygen.)

- Hit them with the "cool factor" defense: Discuss the humiliation associated with vomiting/hospitalization/fill-in-the-blank.
- Never take any drink from anyone they do not know and trust.
- Stick with friends.
- Tell your child you love them. You may not always like their decisions, but you love them and want them safe and to PLEASE CALL if there is any emergency at all.
- Finally DON'T DRINK ALCOHOL.

Set aside time alone to help initiate conversation. It doesn't have to be super serious. Take your child out for an ice cream, dinner, lunch…whatever. Connect with your child. Talk. This isn't the time for lectures; they need to be informed, educated, and engaged. A teenager is more likely to make a good decision if it is their decision, not their mother's or father's. So, help "guide" them to make good decisions. (Wink.) Ask open-ended questions. Play "what if" with them. Remember, the goal here is to keep them healthy, safe, and alive, not to shame and judge.

Rock On, Mom and Dad!

"Does birth control harm your body?" Female, 10th grade

"How sex actually works." Female, 10th grade

MEDICALLY-SPEAKING:

outsourcing medical knowledge

There's an App for That! Managing your Teen's Health and Wellness

The Society for Adolescent Health and Medicine (SAHM) developed an app called **Thrive**. This app allows parents to be an active participant in their child's health. **Thrive** provides a system to help keep track of a child's medical records. It also offers conversation starters, information addressing issues kids face as they grow through adolescence, and important medical information specific for their age.

As a former school nurse, I believe the ability to keep track of your child's medical records is a super cool feature. One of the most important pieces of advice I gave parents is to copy all medical records and keep them in a handy file before relinquishing them to the school. However, with this app, medical information is at the tip of your fingers. Super convenient. Even though my children are in their 20's, occasionally they need some random medical information—usually vaccine history. Think how easy it would be to pull it up on your phone. Ah, technology.

Establishing Trust Between Healthcare Providers and Young People

The American Academy of Pediatrics (AAP) is suggesting to their doctors that it's a good idea to have condoms available for their adolescent patients. They are trying to prevent STIs and unintended pregnancies. Personally, my thought is…what took you so long?

Condoms? Pediatric office? Seriously?? Well, yes. It may seem if a child is seeing a "kid's doctor" they are not old enough to be having sex, but some kids are having sex in (gulp!) middle school. It sounds scary, but this is why it is so important for healthcare providers caring for your children to have an open mind and an open door when it comes to discussing these issues. Conversations between the adolescent and their healthcare provider are crucial for their health; sexual health being just one aspect. This is also a good time for a medical conversation about drug and alcohol use as well. Heaven knows they have already received the parent/guardian "conversation." (*"Don't do it. It's bad for you. You will die–if not from the drugs or sex, it will be from being grounded in your room with no social media to keep you alive."*) I've had that conversation with my kids. Um…it doesn't work.

Encouraging your adolescent to spend some time alone with the physician (without you listening in on their private conversation) can help establish trust between not only the healthcare provider and your child, but also between you and your child. The message you are giving your child is, "Hey, you are growing up. I trust you and respect you enough to have a personal life that you are responsible for."

Of course, after the check-up, you can go in for the "dig"–but do it gently. Open the door for conversation, but don't force it. We all know how well *that* turns out. I would suggest an opening line like, "Was there anything the doctor talked about that you didn't understand?" or "Did you feel comfortable talking to the doctor?" or "I know the doctor can provide a lot of good information. However, if you have any questions that come to mind after your visit, you can ask me. I know it might be difficult, but I love you and care for you and I am here to help." Just leave it at that. You can try saying, "ARE YOU HAVING SEX??!!" but I can pretty much guarantee *no* one will leave happy after *that* conversation.

You may find that your child will say "it's fine!" right away. He or she is processing the information that was given. However, don't be surprised if later on, out of the blue, they approach you with a random question or comment. Stay cool...like you talk about this stuff all the time. I know you are freaking out inside, but you can freak out later, when they aren't looking. Granted, you can't hide the sweat pouring profusely from your brow, but they probably won't notice. Answer their question to the best of your ability. If you are not sure of the answer, tell them that they asked an excellent question and you will find out the answer. At this age, they pretty much think you don't know much anyway, so that won't prevent them from coming back to you with more questions later on down the road. In fact, they will likely appreciate your honesty.

From personal experience, and from what I learned studying adolescent behavior, it is wise to start encouraging private healthcare provider conversations in early middle school. You are laying the groundwork of trust for future conversations–when the topics may become a little more intense. You are also teaching your child how to be an effective healthcare consumer and personal advocate for their own health and well-being. It will serve them well when they head out to college and you aren't there to help them navigate the medical world. Take little steps at a time. I'm not suggesting you drop them off at the physician's all by themselves. Rather, step out of the exam room for just a few minutes to allow time for the healthcare provider and your child to begin to establish an effective patient-doctor relationship. While you are in the waiting room, take a look around for those condoms—that will start a conversation!

———————

Helping Your Adolescent Navigate Their Health World

Navigating the medical world is a necessary–yet sometimes daunting–adult skill. Before you know it, your "sweet baby" will be off to college or work or travel and into a world of independence. Preparing children to take care of themselves is one of our parental responsibilities. After all, illness is inevitable and knowing how to seek appropriate medical care is crucial to their health and ultimate success in school, work, …and life.

I have participated in a health fair at the local high school for a few years now. Our health community gathers together to exhibit and offer information which educates, informs, and increases awareness of services available to students and their families. The students discover available services that may not have been discussed with parents or their health care providers: STI/HIV testing sites, birth control clinics, mental health services, local hospitals, community-based organizations, nutritional services, fitness experts–they all have something to offer our young people. The health fair is an occasion for our youth to explore their health care options without their mom or dad looking over their shoulders. In fact, it is what I love best about this annual event–the sense of autonomy the students gain as they explore the variety of health services available to them in an open, non-judgmental event.

As caring adults, however, we need to continue the education and guidance for our young people as they manage their health. Here are three important, yet basic, skills that you can encourage which will help your child confidently negotiate the medical world.

1. Pick up the phone.

Towards the end of high school your child should feel comfortable calling the appropriate healthcare facility to make an appointment. I know, I know… It is so much easier to do it yourself–I am guilty of that myself. However, helping your child get over the "I don't know what I'm supposed to say" jitters will give them confidence to communicate with providers when they have no one to depend on but themselves. Before they make that call, review with your child the potential questions the scheduler might ask, such as the reason for the visit and insurance information. Be there to offer moral support–and possibly your credit card number.

2. Know whom to call.

Help them understand the difference between medical specialties so they know whom to call for their medical needs. Usually calling one's primary care physician is the best option, but sometimes a specialist may be necessary. For example, if your daughter is having issues with her menstrual cycle or is interested in going on birth control, a gynecologist might be the best option.

3. Be your own advocate. Know which questions to ask to get the answers you need.

Over the years, you have been modeling patient-doctor interaction while your child quietly observed. As your child grows older, teaching him how to communicate his own needs is the next step in establishing health care autonomy. Encourage your child to write out questions for the health care provider and bring them to the appointment. It is so easy to forget everything that is swirling around in our heads before the appointment. When in the exam room, encourage your child to ask questions. But do not interrupt! Your child is in charge now. As an older high school student, it is time to allow your child to visit the doctor on their own. This enables private conversation between the health care provider and your child...and yes, hopefully they are talking about sex! In fact, do not hesitate to request your healthcare provider talk to your child about sexuality.

Watching our "babies" grow into young adults is both exciting and worrisome. After all, they will *never* take care of themselves like *you* take care of them, right? Actually...they will be fine. You taught them well...now let them take charge of their own health care as they head off into the adult world.

(Don't worry, I know from experience they will call you when they are sick...! They still need you.)

Hey Doc, Talk to Me About Sex

One snowy day while working on my project, I was "researching" by leisurely reading the paper. (Okay, so it wasn't research–we all need a minute to relax, right?) I came across a Chicago Tribune article by Karen Kaplan called "Doctors, teens should talk more about sex, study says" (December 30, 2013).[1] I thought to myself... YESSSS! But then I thought...well, duh.

To summarize the article, a study was published in *The Journal of the American Medical Association* (JAMA) Pediatrics addressing the questions: *Do doctors talk to adolescents about sex? If so, how much time do they spend talking about sex? Do the teens engage in the conversation? Are there certain personality types/genders/ ethnicities of the physician or patient that may or may not encourage conversation?* Apparently, no one has really looked into this before. Obviously, I think this is a very, very cool study.

What did they find?
- About 1/3 of the kids who went in for a check-up had no conversation about sexual health with their doctor.
- For the remaining 2/3's who did have a discussion with the doc, the average time discussing sexual health was about 36 seconds.
- Doctors were more likely to speak to older adolescents about sex than younger patients.[2]

Well, let me offer a personal opinion: I'm not sure I consider (an average of) 36 seconds long enough to really get into the topic

---

1   http://articles.latimes.com/2013/dec/30/science/la-sci-sn-doctors-should-discuss-sex-with-teen-patients-20131230 (2013) Doctors and teenage patients should talk more about sex, study says
2   JAMA Pediatr. Published online December 30, 2013. doi:10.1001/jamapediatrics.2013.4338

sexual health. But that's just me. So essentially, discussion about sexual health is pretty much nonexistent in many doctor offices.

And that's a problem. Talking about sexual health with one's physician or other healthcare provider is imperative, whether the patient is an adult or adolescent. This is the opportunity to find out how to protect yourself against unintended pregnancy, STIs, HIV, birth control methods, vaccinations...you name it. After all, medically-accurate, scientifically-based information *is* found in medical clinics.

The study ends with the question–how can professionals change this?? Needless to say, more studies will be done to answer this question.

A Young Woman's Perspective on Talking to her Doc about Sex

The following is a written interview that explored the conversation between a young woman who was about to venture off to college and her healthcare provider. Her answers are insightful: what might make conversations between a young person and a healthcare provider more effective?

Q: *Tell me about the first time your healthcare provider spoke to you about the topic of sexual health. Who brought it up first—you or your provider? Why was it brought up? How old were you?*

A: For several years, my doctor had asked me if I was sexually active, but he always asked me while a parent was in the room, and I felt uncomfortable telling the truth. It wasn't until my senior year in high school that a nurse practitioner talked to me about my own sexual health in private.

Q: *What was the setting of the conversation? Who spoke with you? Did you feel comfortable? How long did the conversation last?*

A: The nurse and I were both in the exam room, and she asked my mom to leave so she could ask me some questions. She was very funny, and I felt comfortable answering her questions. The conversation was probably around 5-10 minutes long, but she covered a lot of different topics.

Q: *Did you find the advice helpful? Were you already familiar with the information that was shared with you?*

A: I found the advice really helpful. I was surprised by how little I knew. The nurse told me information that was new and surprising.

Q: *Do you recall the information that was shared with you?*
Was it relevant to you in particular, or did it feel like a generic
conversation? Was there an opportunity to ask questions?

A: Most of the information we discussed I was familiar with, but
she also shared some things I had never thought about.
For example, she advised me not to share razors with my friends in
order to avoid the spread of HIV. All of the information about sex,
health, drinking and other topics she covered were very relevant to
me at the time. Although she did ask if I had any questions at the
end, I didn't ask any. I wish I would have.

Q: *Was it a positive experience? Shaming? Is there anything that*
would have made the conversation more effective?

A: It was definitely a positive experience. The nurse never made
me feel shameful. The thing that made the conversation most
effective was the privacy. I could ask or say anything to the nurse,
and I knew it would stay in the exam room.

You "Herd" it Here: Immunizations for College Students

Ah, summer...

June and July we have the scent of freshly-mown grass. Long, delicious, velvety evenings with the sound of buzzing mosquitos in our ear (slap!). Farm fresh fruits and vegetables. Splashing in a nearby sparkling body of water. Laughter and shouts of glee as children frolic late into the evening chasing fireflies.

In August, ongoing ad campaigns show happy-faced, jubilant children eagerly luring us to shop for school supplies. (Sure, that's realistic.) Busy shopping centers with students happily spending parent's money on the coolest back-to-school outfits. School orientations to help quell anxious students' uncertainties about the upcoming year. News reports about vicious disease outbreaks at universities.

Wait, what?

Reports concerning occasional outbreaks of mumps on college campuses often make an appearance on local news stations as students return to school. In-coming students are urged to be vaccinated against this unwelcome virus before gracing the campus with their presence. After all, there are parties to attend, new BFF's to meet, oh, and a little learning to be had as well.

But, really, what are the odds your child will need medical care for these diseases? They've been fine so far, right? Hmmm. Let's have a conversation...

When your gifted and amazing child was born, it was–and still is–required for them to receive a multitude of immunizations, with few exceptions.[3] It seemed like every couple of months you routinely bundled up Junior and dragged him/her/other to the doctor for yet another round of pin-cushion practice. Of course, it was always worth it to hear the healthcare providers gush about the unique beauty of your precious one. But deep down, the urgent cries of the most important being in your world were a wee bit distressing.

I trust your child has been given the vaccines necessary for elementary and high school attendance.[4] Most schools will not allow them in the building if they have not received them. I used to be the friendly school nurse who would make the agonizing phone call to busy parents notifying them their child must be picked up from school—on the very first day—due to noncompliance. There were a lot of sad faces, and not just on the parents.

There's this thing called herd immunity.

Let's say you do not feel your child is at risk for a particular disease. You have heard some strange and scary rumors that if your child is given a certain vaccine, their hair will turn purple and their nose will fall off. My suggestion is to not believe everything you hear and read on the internet—including celebrity and other talking head endorsements . Know your sources of information, know the science, talk to your physician.

---

3   http://www.cdc.gov/vaccines/parents/downloads/parent-ver-sch-0-6yrs.pdf (2016)2016 Recommended Immunizations for Children from Birth Through 6 Years Old

4   http://www.cdc.gov/vaccines/who/teens/downloads/parent-version-schedule-7-18yrs.pdf (2016) Information for Parents:2016 Recommended Immunizations for Children 7-18 Years Old

Are all vaccines always risk-free? Of course not. Check out the number of reported side-effects and investigate exactly what those effects are.[5] Trust me on this one—the disease hurts worse than the immunization. Having said that—*always* talk with your doctor. Your child may have some underlying health concern for which a vaccine could have a negative impact on their health. These situations are very rare, but they *do* need to be addressed with your healthcare provider.

With herd immunity, the idea is to vaccinate as many people in the population as possible so that the transmission of disease will not become prolific. Some individuals have health issues and cannot benefit from vaccines. These individuals are depending on the healthy population to become vaccinated so diseases are unable to take hold in communities. When you vaccinate yourself and your children, you are helping prevent nasty diseases such as small pox from resurfacing. In other words, you are being a responsible and admirable citizen of the world and teaching your child to do the same. (Applause)

But, you question, there haven't been (insert any disease here) outbreaks in years! Why should we continue to vaccinate ourselves?

Guess *why* there have not been outbreaks of (the inserted disease) in years? VACCINES.

World travel to all corners of the earth has contributed to the spread of diseases that have been nearly eradicated, such as small pox and polio. Not all countries have such extensive and readily available immunization programs or requirements. If a few unvaccinated or infected people visit from another country, or we visit them…whoosh! We have an outbreak among unvaccinated people. Remember the measles outbreak? Ebola?

---

5   http://www.cdc.gov/vaccines/vac-gen/side-effects.htm (2016) Possible Side Effects from Vaccines

Yeah, I thought so. If there was an Ebola vaccine, would you ask for it? Probably. However, there is a flu vaccine available yet most people do not bother even though it causes more deaths each year than Ebola.[6] (Pause here to contemplate what you just read.)

The vaccinations your child needs as they embark on their future as (sorta) adults in the college world include, but are not limited to, the immunizations listed below.[7]

MMR: Measles, Mumps, Rubella

This immunization is given a couple times, at one year of age and then around kindergarten. However, college kids need to make sure they still have immunity against measles, mumps, and rubella. If not, they need a couple more shots–about 28 days apart. This is the immunization U of I is urgently requesting students check into before school starts–so hurry up.

Let's break it down.

Measles:[8]

- Highly contagious virus
- Lives up to 2 hours after being spewed from a body by coughing, sneezing, etc
- Contagious four days before and four days after the rash appears
- If not immunized there is a 90% chance, after exposure, that you, too will become ill.
- You will become very, very sick. No parties for you.

---

6   http://www.livescience.com/47340-viruses-scarier-than-ebola.html (2014) 5 Viruses that are Scarier than Eobla

7   https://www.vaccines.gov/who_and_when/college/index.html (2016) College and Young Adults

8   http://www.cdc.gov/measles (2015) Measles (Rubeola)

Mumps:[9]

- Highly contagious virus
- Spread by coughing, sneezing, touching, and even talking (Did you know we spew saliva when we talk?)
- Contagious before glands appear swollen and up to 5 days after
- You will become very, very sick. No parties for you.

Rubella (German Measles):[10]

- Virus
- Rash, fever, swollen glands, can affect an unborn baby
- Spread by coughing and sneezing (See a pattern here?)
- You may become very, very sick. (About half do not show symptoms, but they still share the virus.) No parties for you.

Clearly, if you want a guaranteed way to prevent your kids from partying, not being immunized may work. However, you might become a caregiver—which means no parties for you, either, Mom and Dad.

HPV Vaccine: (Gardasil and Cervarix)

The HPV virus, or Human Papillomavirus, is spread by engaging in sex–any kind of sex: oral, vaginal, anal... It can cause cancer, especially cervical and throat.[11] Also warts. On the genitals. There are lots of strains of HPV, but our dedicated researchers have come up with a couple vaccines to decrease the odds of people suffering from these ailments.

---

9 http://www.cdc.gov/mumps (2016) Mumps
10 http://www.cdc.gov/rubella (2016) Rubella
11 http://www.cdc.gov/hpv (2016) Human Papillomavirus (HPV)

For guys, girls, people who identify as neither or both…there is a series of two to three vaccines that should be given around the age of 11-ish.[12] (We need to catch them before they are sexually active, otherwise it may be too late.) I will be honest, a lot of people complain it hurts around the injection site. But seriously, get over it. It is better than the genital warts and cancer. It may be hard for parents to believe that their child may have sex in college. Or ever. And you may be correct. (I'm silently laughing.) Be on the safe side, and start working on the series of three injections to keep your child healthy.

Meningitis[13]

There are a few different vaccines for meningitis, depending on the culprit. Talk to your healthcare provider to discuss the options. Usually students have been vaccinated by high school, but check to make sure your child is. In fact, they probably won't let your child into college without it.

Meningitis is fast-moving and deadly. It is an inflammation of the meninges, a protective layer surrounding the brain. Bacterial meningitis is the most serious, but with a quick diagnosis and antibiotics, there is a cure.

Highly contagious. Spread by coughing, sneezing, kissing, sharing stuff… yawn…you know the drill.

Hepatitis B[14]

Hepatitis B causes liver damage, which isn't fun. It is spread through blood and body fluids. So if your daughter wants to borrow the razor of her roommate for a quick "touch up" and knicks herself…RISK!

---

12 https://www.cancer.gov/about-cancer/causes-prevention/risk/infectious-agents/
    hpv-vaccine-fact-sheet#q5 (2016)Human Papillomavirus (HPV) Vaccines
13 http://www.cdc.gov/meningitis/index.html (2016) Meningitis
14 http://www.cdc.gov/hepatitis/hbv/bfaq.htm (2016)Hepatitis B FAQs for the
    Public

Not everyone has symptoms…but that doesn't mean the virus isn't doing its damage. It only means you don't know who is spreading it.

Tdap

Tdap stands for tetanus, diphtheria, and pertussis.[15] It is likely your child has already had this vaccination to attend school, but a booster of Tdap is to be given every ten years. Yes, even for you Mom and Dad.

- **Tetanus (Lock-Jaw):** Caused by a bacteria entering wounds, basically. It causes muscles to tighten.[16] Example: your non-partying child stepping on an old beer can.
- **Diphtheria:** Bacteria spread by coughing and sneezing. Causes difficulty breathing due to a thick vicious coat on the back of the throat.[17] Yes, and you can die from it–breathing has been scientifically proven to keep humans alive.
- **Pertussis (Whooping Cough):** This one is really making a comeback as well. Caused by a bacteria which causes fits of coughing. This coughing is so intense a person cannot get air into their lungs–when they finally do, it sounds like a "whoop."[18] And not a joyous one either.

Flu Vaccine[19]

This is for everyone including you, Mom and Dad.

Some people mistakenly believe that the "flu shot" protects against something commonly referred to as the "stomach flu." However, as Caitlin E. Cook, MPH (who specializes in infectious disease and

---

15 http://www.cdc.gov/vaccines/parents/diseases/teen/tdap.html (2016) For Parents: Vaccines for Your Children
16 http://www.cdc.gov/tetanus/about/index.html (2013) About Tetanus
17 http://www.cdc.gov/diphtheria/about/index.html (2016) About Diptheria
18 http://www.cdc.gov/pertussis/about/index.html (2016) About Pertussis
19 http://www.cdc.gov/flu (2016) Influenza (Flu)

vaccinology) stated, "People generally misuse the term 'stomach flu.' The illness they are referring to is very rarely caused by influenza virus, and is an unrelated illness. Influenza virus—the true 'flu'—most commonly causes headache, fever, and cough—and generally not nausea and vomiting."

We are talking about the knock-down, drag out, in-bed-for-two-weeks kind of illness. Just ask my brother, who pinky promised me (well, not really) that he will get the flu shot this year after being dragged through the dark days of influenza last year. This can be a very deadly illness. It kills 36,000 people every year and 200,000 are hospitalized according to *Harvard Medical School*.[20]

Granted, sometimes you may end up with influenza despite having the vaccine, however it will lessen the duration and severity of the symptoms. Take note, you cannot get the flu from the vaccine. It takes about two weeks for the vaccine to kick in, so if you come down with the virus within two weeks of being poked, you were exposed before you were protected. Yes, you need to be immunized each year because the virus changes every year.

Just do it. It rarely costs more than $20, and often it is free at your neighborhood clinic or drug store. All it takes is a few minutes of your time. According to the CDC, it decreases your chance of needing medical care by 60%.[21] Plus, think about all the good you are doing in the world by offering herd immunity to those who are physically compromised and could *die* if you do not get the shot.

So, there you have it. The list of vaccines your brilliant, college-bound genius should have before they grace the classroom (or party

20 http://www.health.harvard.edu/diseases-and-conditions/10-flu-myths (2009) 10 Flu Myths
21 http://www.cdc.gov/flu/pdf/freeresources/general/flu-vaccine-benefits.pdf (2016) What are the benefits of flu vaccination?

house) with their presence. Saying goodbye to your child as they head off to college can be difficult. Taking precautions to enhance their health now and in the future will allow you to sleep better at night and know that they are healthy and having fun. Maybe a little too much fun.

Always talk with your healthcare provider about your child's special health concerns.

Hey! It's Not My Fault! It's My Hormones!

Hormones pretty much run our body. Basically, hormones are chemicals that send messages through our body telling it what to do–things like making sure our body is growing, making sure our cells are metabolizing energy, regulating our moods, and even encouraging us to have sex (well, not *all* the time). We have many hormones running through our body that are released from endocrine glands located all over our bodies. But when it comes to the sex hormones, we are primarily talking about the pituitary gland, the hypothalamus, and the gonads.

In a nutshell, the pituitary gland is an endocrine gland about the size of a teeny tiny pea-sized speck in our brain. It is the boss endocrine gland, known as the "master gland." It tells all the other glands what to do and when. A pretty significant little speck, I'd say. Goes to show, bigger *isn't* always better!

The hypothalamus, also in the brain, is located just above the pituitary. We all know how important communication is in a relationship and this is no different. In fact, it's essential. This guy takes care of things we don't really think about–things that happen automatically. It regulates our heart beats, our body temperature, our respirations, and thirst and hunger. It also regulates sex drive and produces some sex hormones. We really like this part of the brain.

Finally, there are the gonads. In men they are the testes, and in women they are the ovaries. These guys are the primary producers of the hormones we will discuss. We kinda like these parts, too.

These three seemingly independent parts of the body work in tandem with each other, constantly communicating. If one hormone is a little low or a little high, an alert is sent out by the hypothalamus to the pituitary, which then sends a message to the gonad to adjust the hormonal input or output.

A classic comparison of how this works is similar to how the heating system in your home operates. You have a set point you prefer to keep your home comfortable. Let's say it's 73 degrees. When the thermostat senses that it is now 72 in the house, it kicks on until it reaches 73 again. However, when it reaches 74, it shuts off. Fairly well regulated. Our body does the same thing with hormones. The hypothalamus and pituitary know what we need to function optimally, and when it senses a sex hormone is a little off, it sends messages to the correct gland to fix it.

There are many essential hormones required to maintain sexual health. However, we will focus on the three we hear the most about; testosterone, estrogen, and progesterone. Whether a person is male, female, or intersex, they will have all three hormones in their system. They are all essential. However, depending on one's gender, there are more of some than others.

Testosterone we consider a male hormone, and it is. But we all need it to build muscle and bone. In guys, the testes produce it. In gals, it's the ovaries. Around puberty, guys produce a lot more of it and girls slow down their production, thanks to estrogen. Testosterone helps boys become men by increasing their bulk, growing pubic and facial hair, lowering their voice, and increasing the need for deodorant, among other changes. (These are called secondary sex characteristics.) It is also instrumental in sexual desire and sperm production, which takes place in the testes.

Estrogen is actually an umbrella term for different kinds of estrogen; estriol, estradiol, and estrone. But estrogen is the term typically used for simplicity. This hormone helps make little girls into women:

hair growth, womanly figure, breast development, and reproductive organ growth and development. (These are also called secondary sex characteristics.) Estrogen also helps regulate the menstrual cycle and helps prepare the body for pregnancy. This, too, is largely produced in the ovaries, but males produce small amounts in the testes.

Progesterone is another (primarily female) hormone predominately produced in both gonads. This hormone helps us feel sexy, helps regulate the menstrual cycle, and helps prepare and maintain the uterus during pregnancy. You may have heard of progestin as well. I want to point out that this is actually a synthetic, or man-made, hormone similar to progesterone.

So, now you know. But to summarize……..

Hormones: Chemical messengers
Pituitary Gland: In the brain. Master gland–gives all the orders.
Hypothalamus: In the brain. Regulates things that happen automatically but also produces sex hormones.
Gonads: The sex organs that produce hormones. Testes in males and ovaries in females. The testes produce sperm, and the ovaries produce eggs (ova).
Testosterone: Gives guys their sex characteristics, encourages sex drive, and helps produce sperm.
Estrogen: Gives gals their sex characteristics, helps regulate monthly cycle, and maintains the reproductive organs.
Progesterone: Prepares body for pregnancy, helps regulate monthly cycle.

Puberty...A Time for Perfecting the Eyeball Roll

What happens to our precious, loving, adorable, little children? Where do they go when they hit about 11 or 12 years old? Will they ever return to us as they were just a few short months/years ago?

I can tell you from experience...yes. Yes they will. But having a grasp at what is causing their eyeballs to roll uncontrollably–and what you can do to keep your sanity–oh, I mean be there for your child–can help these fascinating adolescent years become a memorable experience...and I mean that in the best sense.

When our wee ones grow into young children, they pretty much think we are amazing. Whatever we say is true and real. ("Yes, Honey, Mommy *does* have naturally blond hair.") And they actually want to do stuff with us. ("Dad, can we go see a movie today?")

But in early childhood, before we can even see the stirrings of puberty, underneath that sweet exterior, something sinister is happening...hormones are revving up. The pituitary gland, the gland that pretty much bosses all the other glands around, starts sending meaningful signals to a few key reproductive glands.

The first gland to be hit by these signals is the adrenal gland. This guy starts sending out hormones which begin the process of change. A few years later, the real fun begins when the pituitary tells the testes and ovaries to do their thing–release testosterone and estrogen, respectively–initiating P-U-B-E-R-T-Y.

How do we know when these changes are going to occur? We don't really, but we can make a pretty educated guess.

Briefly, genetics are a significant factor–how old were you when you started puberty? The environment factors in as well. Stress level, access to adequate health care, nutrition, and family environment can all impact the onset of puberty, especially when considering the start of a young girl's menstrual cycle.

But what the heck is going on inside their heads? Well, it's really not as bad as you think. There are a lot of studies that can be found about the psychological processes within the brains of adolescents. Apparently, a lot of researchers have raised adolescent children and wanted answers as well. So, here is a little information you may find helpful.

Snarkiness, I mean puberty, may begin in girls at about age 9 or as late as 15. In boys, it typically begins between 12-16. These changes start to affect their self-esteem. They wonder if they are developing too early–or too late. They start comparing themselves to other kids, especially the girls. This is demonstrated in the ad when she brags to all her "blood sisters" that she is finally in the "cherry slush club." She doesn't want to be different. She wants to go through this rite of passage with her BFF's.

As their bodies are changing and hormones are dancing around, their school environment and social circles begin to evolve, too. Moving from grade school to middle school, where they are introduced to a new gathering of pubescent humans, they need to reestablish themselves in a comfortable group of friends–which takes time. It's pretty stressful–even for an adult. That would make anyone cranky.

How many have heard their kids say, "You don't understand!"? Yup. I thought so. All of you. Early adolescents pretty much center their thinking around themselves. They feel as if no one has ever "felt like this" before. ("You don't know what it feels like to be in loooveeeee like this, Mom!") They assume that everyone is looking at them, like when they trip over a twig or have a bad hair day. They also believe "it won't happen to me." (This one scares me the most: "I won't get pregnant.") The good news is, they will grow out of it eventually.

Another interesting find is these delightful adult-wanna-be's tend to be most crabby around adults, not so much around their peers. (No kidding, right?) The structure and expectations adults set on them kind of stresses them out a bit. And the reason their moods fluctuate so often? Because between school and activities, they flip-flop between adults (who sometimes annoy them) and peers (who usually delight them) so much more frequently.

Yes, as our kids start going through these life-altering changes, they do tend to become moody, less lovey-dovey, hide in their room more often, argue a bit more...and want to hang with their friends rather than you. (What? You're going to the movies *with* me? You're ruining my life!")

That's okay. You know why? They are starting to form their own identity and are learning how to navigate some independence...and that's a wonderful thing. But we'll talk about that another time.

In the meantime, what can you do? Well, as I've said before, just be there. Give them some room to grow as a person. Discuss and set reasonable boundaries and expectations with them. Have them be part of the conversation–it will communicate to them that their thoughts and opinions are valued and respected. (Be sure to follow through on the agreed upon discipline if they choose to break the rules.) Be interested in their lives. They may blow you off, but trust me–it matters to them that you care enough to ask and to show up at their activities. Try to spend some alone time with them. It builds a foundation of closeness and trust for future conversations.

Just as important, take care of yourself! We all need a little time to decompress. So, call a friend and grab a glass of wine or beer, a piece of chocolate, a freshly baked cupcake, whatever it is that helps calm your soul. (Oh, wait, I'm a health teacher. Call a friend and go for a walk while eating a banana.) Not only does it do you good mentally, but you will model healthy ways to cope with daily stress.

Interestingly, a worldwide study was done about adolescents and their relationship with their parents. From Bangladesh to the USA it was found, overwhelmingly, our kids actually love us and know we love them. They also respect our values and advice.

So, you see? It's really not that bad. Just a little bumpy here and there. I've been through it three times and have survived the roller-coaster myself. Trust me, those sweet little innocent angels are no longer, but rather have been replaced with some pretty remarkable and kind young adults that enjoy spending time with me–and I with them!

Resource for this information is the textbook:

Kail, Robert V., and John C. Cavanaugh. "Chapter 8-9." Human Development: A Life-span View. Australia: Thomson/Wadsworth, 2007. N. pag. Print.

Let's Talk: Cervical Health

January is National Cervical Health Awareness Month.

So, let's talk cervix....

The cervix is part of the female reproductive system. It is a couple inches long and is connected to the uterus and vagina. It has a very small opening–the cervical os, that allows menstrual flow to exit the body. Even more remarkable, it stretches wide enough to allow a full-sized baby to slide into the world. When a woman is in labor, the healthcare providers will assess the readiness of a woman's body to deliver by measuring the dilation of the cervix. The nurse or doctor will frequently perform internal exams to evaluate the diameter of the cervical os using a scale of 1 to 10 centimeters. When it is a "10", it is time to PUSH!

Unless your gynecologist whipped out a speculum and a mirror for your educational entertainment, you probably have not actually seen your cervix. Therefore, it is difficult for women to visualize and assess if something unhealthy is brewing. In addition, cervical cancer is often silent; there are no obvious signs and symptoms. This is why it is recommended to visit your healthcare provider on an annual basis.

According to the National Cervical Cancer Coalition, cancer of the cervix is diagnosed in about 12,000 U.S. women each year.[22] Four thousand die. Globally, it is the second most common cancer among women. It is a highly preventable and treatable cancer when suggested health guidelines are followed.

22 http://www.nccc-online.org/hpvcervical-cancer/cervical-health-awareness-month (2016) Cervical Cancer Overview

Signs and Symptoms of Cervical Cancer

- Abnormal bleeding
- Abdominal pain
- Unusual discharge
- Painful sex
- Painful urination or increase in bathroom breaks

These symptoms indicate any of a number of health issues, which is why a visit to your provider is necessary when you experience unusual manifestations.

Tests

The Pap smear is a swab sample of your cervix to detect any cancerous or pre-cancerous cells present.[23] Since the introduction of Pap smears in the 50's, cancer rates in the U.S. have dropped about 60% among women of child-bearing age.[24]

HPV screening involves a swab sample of your cervix as well, often at the same time as the Pap test.[25] This screening is different, however, because it detects the DNA of human Papillomavirus (HPV). HPV is the virus that causes cervical cancer. Recent research indicates that HPV testing be the primary screening for cervical cancer rather than the Pap smear. However, the combination of the two offers invaluable information to your provider.

---

23 http://www.ashasexualhealth.org/making-sense-pap-tests-hpv-tests-new-landscape-cervical-cancer-screening (2016) Making Sense of Pap Tests, HPV Tests, and the New Landscape of Cervical Cancer Screening

24 https://report.nih.gov/nihfactsheets/viewfactsheet.aspx?csid=76 (2013) Cervical Cancer

25 http://www.nccc-online.org/hpvcervical-cancer/cervical-cancer-screening/ (2016) Cervical Cancer Screening: Pap and HPV Tests

A woman may have a negative Pap and positive HPV test, Positive Pap and negative HPV, or both negative or both positive.

Treatment

Depending on the result, your healthcare provider will suggest treatment; often a wait-and-see approach is taken. This type of pre-cancerous cell grows slowly, so waiting a few months or a year to see if the test results are different is pretty standard. However, your provider might suggest removing the questionable cells with a follow-up procedure shortly thereafter. It all depends on the test results and what your provider observes during exam.

Prevention

Regular visits to your healthcare provider for screening are invaluable. Identifying and removing rogue cells early will save your life.

Screening Guidelines:

- Beginning at age 21, women should have a Pap smear every three years until approximately age 65. Older women, even if sex is not a part of their current lifestyle, should continue to be tested as cervical cancer may present itself two decades after exposure to HPV.
- Up to age 30, a pap smear every 3 years is all that is necessary, depending on personal medical history and doctor's recommendation.
- After age 30, an HPV screening test and Pap smear may be used together to screen women for cervical cancer. If both tests are negative, the next screening is typically at five years.
- Alternatively, if only an HPV screening is done, it should be repeated every three years, much like the Pap smear.

Confused? Don't be. Talk to your healthcare provider to come up with a plan that works with your comfort level and medical history. The days of annual Pap smears are over, however, so do not fret when providers suggest waiting a few years in between tests, but not exams.

Dr. Carolyn Mills, an obstetrician and gynecologist at Dreyer Medical Clinic in the Chicago suburbs, recommends women not neglect their annual gynecological exam between HPV and Pap screenings. As a vagina-owner, how often are you able to spend an hour or so talking about yourself, uninterrupted, about your most personal health issues? An annual exam is an excellent opportunity to talk with your healthcare provider about ongoing issues regarding contraception, breast health, and reproductive health. Additionally, there are other reproductive health issues that may be caught early by the health professional. For example, STIs in general do not always present with symptoms; taking the time to give your healthcare provider an honest sexual history is imperative to receiving the excellent care every woman deserves.

On a personal note, I have always scheduled my exams during the month of May, the month I celebrate my birthday. Why? It is easy to remember, but honestly, what better gift can a person give themselves than the gift of good health? Well, shoes. There's that, too. Take a "Me Day" and visit your gynecologist, your favorite shoe store, and perhaps lunch with a friend during your birthday month. In one glorious day a woman can address her physical, mental/emotional, and social wellness needs.

Vaccinations:

The HPV vaccine was introduced within the last decade.[26] This vaccine prevents the specific strains of HPV that cause cancer (cervical, anal, penis, oral) and genital warts from taking hold. At the age of 11 or 12, boys and girls are able to receive the HPV vaccine. This immunization is a series of two to three injections over the course of six months.[27] The key is to vaccinate children before they become sexually active and are exposed to HPV. This vaccine is approved to be given up to the age of 26; if a person only received one or two injections of the series of three, they are able to finish out the regimen as a young adult. The vaccines are Gardasil 9, and Cervarix. However, even with the coverage the vaccine offers, it is not 100% effective. It is necessary to continue with your Pap smears and/or HPV tests.

Cervical cancer used to be a leading cause of death among women in their child-bearing age. With the introduction of the Pap smear in the 1950's, that number decreased about 60% according to the National Institute of Health.[28] However, despite health care professionals' best efforts, it is the number two cancer among women worldwide. In the U.S., with the introduction of HPV screenings and the HPV vaccine, those numbers are expected to decline rapidly. Continue to visit your healthcare provider on a regular basis and discuss with them your plan of action to help prevent this treatable and preventable cancer.

───────────────

26 http://www.cdc.gov/vaccines/parents/diseases/teen/hpv.html (2015) HPV Vaccine for Preteens and Teens
27 http://www.cdc.gov/media/releases/2016/p1020-hpv-shots.html (2016) CDC recommends only two HPV shots for younger adolescents
28 https://report.nih.gov/nihfactsheets/viewfactsheet.aspx?csid=76 (2013) Cervical Cancer

A Journey with Marcy: Cervical Cancer

Have you ever met someone who lights up a room merely by their presence? Someone for whom it seems no matter what life throws at them, they keep their chin up, keep a smile on their face, and breezily deal with the issues life presents?

I would like you to meet a friend of mine for over a decade. Marcy Zirbel is a 50 year-old mother of two delightful daughters. Several years ago, thanks to her annual Pap test, she was diagnosed with early stage cervical cancer. She is very happy to share her medical journey with other women to be a source of information and inspiration.

Marcy we know that cervical cancer is very difficult to diagnose. Would you share with us how you found out you had cervical cancer?

I was just 36 when I was diagnosed through my yearly PAP test. We were new to the Chicagoland area, and it was the first time I had seen this particular Ob-Gyn, who I picked out of my insurance company directory because she was a woman. Her office called me to say that the PAP showed severe dysplasia, and they scheduled a colposcopy about a week later. I had undergone a colposcopy before in my 20's, so I was not worried.

Would you explain what a colposcopy is?

Certainly. During the procedure, the doctor dyes the cervix to see the areas of abnormal cells. She identified 2 areas of concern on the surface of the cervix and biopsied both of them. The biopsies confirmed the dysplasia, so they scheduled me for a "LEEP" procedure to remove the two areas, and I was still not concerned. On the day of the "LEEP" (I drove myself there and probably shouldn't have, but my ex-husband was absent), the Ob-Gyn decided at the last minute to use a cone shaped wire to grab a bigger sample and go deeper into the cervix where they couldn't see.

When the doctor personally called me about 6 days later, I was shocked to hear that she said I had Stage 1B cervical cancer and she referred me to a Gynecological Oncologist. She said, "I know that you probably didn't hear anything after I said the "C" word, so after you digest the news, you may call me back later tonight with questions.

Wow, so it sounds like you had a terrific physician. When you were diagnosed, did your doctor explain how women "get" cervical cancer?

Neither the first doctor, nor my oncologist, volunteered any opinion of how they thought I got it. I immediately began researching on the Internet to inform myself, and the thinking at the time was that young women contract the HPV virus in their 20's and it can lie dormant for years and sometimes come out later in life.

I see. That must have added additional stress to an already frightening situation. At that point, what was the treatment protocol your doctor suggested?

My Gyne-Oncologist is the most wonderful, humble, caring man. He was not an alarmist at all and told me in my initial visit that a radical hysterectomy would be curative. Since I was so young, he left my ovaries, but tacked them out of the way in case he needed to follow up with radiation in the future. Chemotherapy was never mentioned, which was a relief in my mind. I also spoke to a cousin and friend who are doctors, and they both agreed that if you are going to get cancer, cervical is the one to get because it is 100% curable if caught early, like mine.

How fortunate you take care of your body and visit your healthcare provider for cervical cancer screenings. It saved your life.
We talked about the physical aspect of cervical cancer, however it must take a toll mentally and emotionally. Can you talk a little about that?

My girls were so little when I was diagnosed (4 & 8) that the only thing I could think was, "I can't leave these two perfect little girls without a mom." I stopped reading about cervical cancer on the Internet about 24 hours after I found out because all the "what-ifs" can drive you crazy. I decided to stay positive and thankful...I really believe in the mind-body connection.

My best friend said, "I don't understand it. You don't drink or smoke, you exercise and eat all the right things. If this could happen to you..." I never walked around with a negative, "why me?" attitude. I stayed positive and focused on healing.

How about now? How are you mentally/emotionally with this diagnosis now that you have been given a clean bill of health?

I don't even think about it anymore (14 years later). I saw my oncologist every 3 months for the first 2 years, and then every 6 months for the next 3 years. After the 5-year clear mark, he told me I had "graduated" to the one year plan for PAP tests and internal exams. But he said that if I was worried about waiting a year to see him, please just come in and he would find a way to make the insurance cover it. I am so thankful to have survived! I just got married this summer, and my husband's first wife of 27 years died of cancer. I think we were meant to find each other.

I believe people come into your lives for a reason. I am certain you were meant to find each other. You have two daughters, 18 and 22. From a cervical cancer survivor's perspective and as a mom, what is your perspective on preventative immunizations such as Gardasil?

I am all for immunizing both girls and boys with Gardasil. I think it's been on the market for at least 10 years now, and they routinely offer it at the pediatrician's office and insurance covers it. .

That is correct. How would you respond to parents who are understandably hesitant because of their concerns about the immunization? Typical concerns revolve around the safety of the medication, unknown future effects of the immunization, and also the fear that giving their child this immunization will encourage them to become sexually active.

I think that parents need to educate themselves about HPV and Gardasil, just like with all vaccines. When we were children, the small pox vaccine was routinely given to everyone. Now small pox has basically been eradicated, and there is no need to vaccinate our children. Likewise, when my older daughter was about 5, our pediatrician offered the chicken pox vaccine. I elected to give it to both her and my 1 year old at the same time. It was rather new back then, and many friends were not vaccinating their kids, but instead saying chicken pox was not so bad. A lot was not known about the varicella vaccine 17 years ago, like how long it would last or if a booster would be required. In fact, the varicella vaccine is now required for students to attend school, at least in Illinois. I am confident that the HPV vaccine can evolve in the same way.

Suffering from cervical cancer is not even in the same universe as suffering with chicken pox. Giving the HPV vaccine to young girls and boys as a standard vaccination (recommended as young as 11) takes the sexual component out of the equation.

Thank you so much for your time, Marcy. You have provided a thoughtful and honest reflection about your experience with cervical cancer. Is there anything you would like to add that you feel parents, educators, and health care providers should understand from the perspective of a mother and a cervical cancer survivor?

It makes me happy to be able to share my experience to help others, and I believe a positive attitude is everything. When I was in the hospital after my hysterectomy, one of my nurses came up to me at the end of her shift and said that I was totally different than she expected when she read my chart. She went on to say that she had the same thing when she was 28, and she was not married and had no children. She said that seeing how grateful and cheerful I was helped her...and here I had been thanking her all day for helping me!

I had two beautiful girls and did not want any more kids, so when they told me a hysterectomy would cure my cancer, I said, "Take it out!" Now my oldest daughter is in her third year of pharmacy school, and she said what I lived through inspired her to want to help others, too.

Marcy, you have certainly inspired your daughters. You have also inspired me with your positive spirit and forthright honesty. Thank you for your time and thoughts. It is greatly appreciated.

For more information about cervical heath, go to the National Cervical Cancer Coalition.-

11 Ways to Avoid Colds and Flu

This morning as I was lying in bed, thinking about blogging, work, projects, plans, shopping…you know…all that stuff that keeps us up at night, my mind drifted to the current state of affairs in my world. No, not the increased violence both globally and nationally. (What the heck is going on, people??) No, not the fear of global warming. No, not the alarm about catastrophic earthquakes poised to hit California. Rather…colds and flu.

This has nothing to do with adolescent sexual health, other than being sick could be a deterrent for anyone to engage in sex. However, as a nurse, health educator, and someone who has studied public health, I could not pass up this opportunity to educate about simple ways to help prevent the spread of cold and flu viruses. Both colds and flu can knock a person down, but the flu is worse: Secondary infections are severe and can require hospitalization–about 200,000 a year, in fact.*

---

* Secondary infections are infections a person may get due to the havoc caused by the flu virus. Typically seen in people who are elderly or who are immunocompromised (unable to fight off illness like the rest of us). This is why the flu vaccine is highly encouraged for certain populations.

The good news is that once you have a certain virus, you are immune to it for life. That bad news is viruses are constantly changing, and there are countless ones out there. You won't be immune to those unless you suffer through the effects of that particular strain or are vaccinated. And there is no "cold vaccine" out there yet. However, there is a flu vaccine. I get mine every year. No brainer. It's usually free with insurance or never more than 20 bucks. It only takes a few minutes at your local doc-in-a-box.

Many people choose not to get the vaccine, despite the affordability and convenience. The most common excuses I hear include: "I don't need the vaccine," "the vaccine doesn't work," or "I always get sick when I get the vaccine.

Maybe they do not need the vaccine. Who am I to say? Some people don't mind taking the risk of becoming ill. And if they do become sick, they just deal with it for a week or two then move on. Personally, that's a week of hell I'd rather avoid. Been there, done that.

As far as the vaccine not working, well each year the CDC has to decide which strain of the flu is the one that will cause havoc. It's a guessing game, but a very educated guess based on what's going on in Asia. Sometimes it's right on, sometimes it's a miss. However, even if it's a 'miss," the vaccine will still protect you from becoming severely ill if you become sick. It will help lessen the symptoms. And if it's a hit, you may avoid the entire mess all together.

No, the vaccine does not cause the flu. If you get the vaccine then become ill afterwards, that merely means you received the vaccine too late–you were already exposed to the virus. Just dumb luck. It takes about two weeks for the vaccine to kick in.

This is not to say some people can't have an allergic reaction to the vaccine, but it is extremely rare. The healthcare provider will take your medical history to assess your risk, and do not hesitate to discuss any concerns with your provider.

Prevention is best.

No one is a hero when they come to work sick. You are not superwoman or superman because you can continue to function with a fever, headache, and body aches. Think about how many people just one person can infect. Not only have they shared the virus with their own family, but now their co-workers and their families have been exposed. If the business is client-based, each client that has walked in the door has now been exposed and will then unknowingly bring the virus back to their families and co-workers. Please. Break the chain. Keep in mind a person is typically contagious one day before symptoms appear and up to 5 days after the onset of the illness began.

Once you are ill, it's okay to rest. I have always said it's my body's way of telling me to *slow down*. (Plus, a little movie-time is good for the soul, don't you think?)

Here are some simple steps to help prevent the spread of colds and flu:

1. Wash your hands. With soap and water. Just rinsing with water is *not* washing your hands. I don't mean wash your hands just once when you wake up. I don't mean only after you use the bathroom. (You *do* wash your hands after you use the bathroom, don't you?) I don't mean just occasionally. I mean when you blow your nose or touch any bodily fluid–yours or another person's (like your child's runny nose), wash your hands with soap and water. Antibacterial gels are okay in a pinch, but soap and water is the best. As a rule of thumb, scrub your hands about 20 seconds to effectively remove the yuck.
2. Avoid touching your mucus membranes (aka: nose, mouth, eyes.) That's like a little viral train depot–they love the moist, warm environment that enables them to take off on their adventure to Body Land.
3. Use disposable paper towels, not hand towels. If hand towels are used, replace or wash them frequently.
4. Dispose of used tissues properly. Don't just throw them on the floor for someone else to pick up.
5. Sneeze in your sleeve (i.e. elbow), not your hand. Doesn't it gross you out when people sneeze in their hands, then

proceed to grab a doorknob, or fresh produce at the grocery store, or shake your hand? Just ewwww. Think about it.

6. Better than an elbow: sneeze in a tissue and dispose of it. Fluid droplets are the primary method of virus-sharing, so stop sneezing in the air.

7. Don't put your grubby hands on food that others will eat. As a general rule of thumb, putting your hand into packaging to retrieve tasty morsels is never a good idea. Don't stick your hand in a bag of chips or popcorn. Don't put your hands in a bowl of M&M's. Rather pour out your serving of chips or popcorn. Use a spoon to retrieve those sweet treats. That's just a general rule of thumb when it comes to food safety anyway; often viruses are being shared before the person even knows they are sick.

8. Disinfect, disinfect, disinfect surfaces. Cold and flu viruses can live on surfaces for up to 8 hours. Death to the germs!

9. Stay home and rest. Duh. The general rule of thumb is to stay away from humanity until you are fever-free (100 degrees or more) for 24 hours. *Without* the aid of medication.

10. Drink lots of fluids and yes, eat chicken soup. It really has been proven to help with congestion, thanks to the warmth and steam.

11. Don't be afraid to ask for help. Years ago, I was down flat with the flu. It was awful. But what made it worse was my three young daughters also had the flu. My husband was on vacation in sunny Florida, while we were hunkered down cozied up trying to feel better. (Do I sound bitter?) I didn't have the energy to prepare a lot of meals, so I called a neighbor and asked if he would mind getting us some food for dinner. It was humbling, but that is what friends are for! I will never forget that kindness. If you have friends who are sick, I suggest bringing them a meal. Try to deliver it by drone so you can avoid the germ-fest. (And send me a video of that delivery–that would be so cool!)

Granted, it is not always easy to do all the suggestions mentioned all the time. But be aware and be considerate of others. Getting your flu vaccine, staying home from work, diligent hand-washing, not touching your eyeballs, or picking your nose and teeth; those are simple steps we can take to prevent others and ourselves from becoming ill.

I have years of experience as an elementary school nurse. There was a funny comic shared with our good-humored nurses that shows a little boy talking to the school nurse saying, "I woke up coughing, with a sore throat, and a fever. My mom said to try and make it through the day." HaHaHa. Okay—I guess you had to be there. Maybe it was just "nurse humor," but trust me, it was funny. The truth is kids are often sent to school exactly like this! Certainly you can't stay home, or keep your kids home, for every little sniffle. That is totally unrealistic. But if learning or working effectively due to illness is an issue, just take the day off.

Now for a personal story of which I am NOT proud. Years ago, when I was a young mom, there was a really great sale at a local department store. I felt awful, but not *so* awful to keep me away from a S-A-L-E! I remember dragging my exhausted body through the store while carting my children around in their stroller. A salesclerk approached me and asked me if I was okay. Apparently, I looked like the wife of Frankenstein. I don't remember how I responded (possibly I was delirious) but she gave me a stern look and told me to go home and get some rest. I guess she told me! But she was right. Whenever I think about venturing out for a non-essential errand when I'm feeling under the weather, I think back to that incident and the wisdom of that crabby salesclerk.

It's our nature as busy adults to keep persevering through hardships. It's the American way! But I am urging you to take care of yourself. Cuddle up with a hot cup of tea, a great movie, your stuffed teddy bear (I won't tell) and just take one day for yourself to try and get better. Your body, your co-workers, your friends, your family will be grateful to you.

Stay Well!

———————

Campaign to Change Direction: Mental Health and Adolescence

Your son used to bound down the stairs each evening and eagerly plant himself between you and your spouse. Chatting about his day, you delighted in hearing about his colorful adventures. But lately he prefers sitting quietly in his room each evening. He says he is doing homework—who can complain about that? Yet you have a feeling something is not quite right. You miss your enthusiastic, fun-loving boy.

Oh, the moody teenage years. Your mother warned you about raising a teenager. However, she failed to mention adolescence can be as difficult for the parent as the child. What is a parent to do? Your daughter flies off the handle for the silliest things. Does putting one's laundry away warrant a screaming match? She used to be so much fun to be around, but lately she seems irritable and angry. Did I do something wrong? Maybe it is just those teenage hormones.

Adolescence is a time of rapid mental, emotional, social, and physical growth. It is a time for exploring one's identity, aspirations, and interests. Watching your child develop into their own person is at the same time exciting and daunting. Mood swings, crabbiness, and irritation can be expected. After all, we all have bad days. But what if it is something more? What if your child is actually experiencing a mental condition that requires treatment? How would you know?

I recently attended a summit about the topic of anxiety and depression among young people. It was presented by a recently launched campaign called the *Campaign to Change Direction*. This organization's mission is to ignite conversation about mental/emotional health and wellness.

By educating the public about five recognizable symptoms, individuals who are quietly suffering may finally get help. The stigma of mental illness may be eliminated by recognizing that mental health is equally important as physical health and that mental health issues are very common. According to *Change Direction*, about one in five individuals have a mental health condition, including depression and anxiety. But more importantly, "HALF of all mental disorders begin by age 14."

Age 14.

In fact, one of the young people on the panel of the summit stated that her problems began about the age of 7.

As I listened to these amazing, brilliant, outstanding young people share their stories, it dawned on me; how many times did I assume a child was just quiet, or shy, or having a bad day, when in fact they may have been dealing with something deeper that deserved recognition? It is so easy to brush people off and attribute moodiness to their personality; sure, maybe it is their disposition–or maybe they need help.

The Campaign to Change Direction offers five signs that indicate a person may need help.

1. Their personality changes. They just seem different from their usual selves. This may happen suddenly or very gradually.
2. They seem unusually irritable, moody, anxious, angry. Little things can set them off, and they may have difficulty sleeping.
3. They withdraw or isolate themselves when they used to be socially engaged. They may no longer attend work or school and may withdraw from teams or clubs they previously enjoyed.
4. They may stop caring for themselves. Their personal hygiene may be lacking or they may not care about their appearance. They may begin to engage in risky behavior such as cutting, drinking or drugging.

5. They may feel hopeless and overwhelmed. They are no longer optimistic. They may feel they do not matter, which may indicate suicidal thoughts.

As parents and friends, what can we do to help individuals struggling with emotional health?

This question was posed to the student panel at the *Change Direction* event. The students stated that the best way to support someone with mental health problems is to simply be there and listen, be supportive and caring. If the situation requires further help, for example if the person talks about harming themselves, get help. Tell a trusted adult and professional, such as a school social worker or psychologist, parent, psychiatrist, or therapist.

Offering solutions, telling them it will all be better, minimizing their feelings, and telling them to "get over it" are not a positive approach. It fact, it could be detrimental. Feeling judged may prevent someone who is suffering from reaching out for professional help.

Treatment is available in the form of counseling and medication. Finding a therapist and psychiatrist that both parent and adolescent trust will enable healing. However mental health is often a life-long condition that requires continued care. Just like many medical conditions. Finding a therapist with whom the child connects is crucial-you may have to "interview" a few to find the right fit.

Reach out to the young person or adult in your life whom you feel may be going through a difficult time. A kind word, a supportive gesture, a quick "how have you been?" can make a tremendous difference to a person who is hurting.

Find *The Campaign to Change Direction* at http://www.changedirection.org.

Kim T. Cook, RN CHES

"What is something that someone can do to be introduced to the proper use of contraception?" Female, 12th grade

"Does pre-cum have sperm?" Female, 11th grade

"Whys other than abstinence not to get pregnant." Female, 12th grade

CONTRACEPTION:

how to prevent early grandparenthood

Condoms: What's Your Pleasure?

Condoms. Rubbers. Raincoats. Sheaths. Love Gloves. Prophylactics. Wetsuits. Willie Warmers.

Condoms. Despite all the fun, slang terms we have for this barrier method of birth control, they are just about the only method we have to prevent STIs and HIV. Wait. That is not a true statement… *Abstinence* is the *only* way to prevent STIs, HIV, and pregnancy. Period. Because most people do in fact have sex, people need to be informed about safer sex practices to reduce the risk of STIs/HIV/pregnancy by using condoms.

For simplicity's sake, I am going to refer to condoms as "male" and "female." However, I want to make clear that I appreciate that some individuals with penises identify as "female," and some people with vaginas identify as "male" and others identify as non-binary.

Now, let's get started with information and talking points you can share with your child.

Male Condoms

- They protect best against STIs transmitted via body fluids. They are not as effective against STIs spread through skin-to-skin contact, such as herpes.
- If a condom is used correctly and consistently–every time a person has sex–it is 98% effective. Unfortunately, most people do not use it every time or they use it incorrectly, so its effectiveness is only about 80-90% as a general rule. (*National Institute of Health* (NIH))[1],[2]
- They come in flavors (you know, the oral thing…) and colors, sizes, and textures.

1   http://www.nlm.nih.gov/medlineplus/ency/article/004001.htm (2015) Condoms - Male
2   http://www.cdc.gov/condomeffectiveness/docs/CondomFactsheetInBrief.pdf Condom Fact Sheet In Brief

- They are made from different materials. These include:

  Latex Rubber: These are the most popular. They help protect against both STIs/HIV and pregnancy. They are pretty inexpensive–about a buck a piece. However, some people are allergic to latex.

  Polyurethane: These protect against both STIs/HIV and pregnancy. Great for people who are allergic to latex. Not as tight-fitting, so some people like these better.

  Sheepskin: Only protects against pregnancy. Because it is made of animal skin, it is porous, therefore those pesky little viruses and bacteria can sneak through the condom. Definitely a great option for a monogamous couple.

- There are many brands. Trojan, Durex, and Lifestlyes are three major players in the condom business. There are many smaller companies as well; sort of like the microbreweries of condoms. Some of these brands have donated their condoms to various organizations for free distribution, so kudos to them.

- They are inexpensive. About $1 to $4 a piece, depending on the brand, place of purchase, or material it is made from. (A *whole* lot cheaper than antibiotics and babies.)

- Before using a condom, check the expiration date. If it is expired, do not use it. Would you drink expired wine? I thought not. Consume expired chocolate? Oh, wait. Bad example.

- Do not store condoms in really cold or really hot places. Room temp, please.

- If a person stores a condom in their wallet, their body heat and frequent movement increases the risk of damage to the package. Rotate it out frequently. Fresh is best!

- Make sure the condom package is not deflated. If it is, there is probably a hole in the packaging…and maybe in the condom.

- Put the condom on *before* your sexy bits touch your partner's sexy bits. Otherwise, you've defeated the purpose; pre-cum has little swimmers that are eager to find their target.

- Use one every time you have sex, and use it correctly. Read the directions and practice.
- Do not reuse. This is one time where reusing and recycling is a very, very bad idea.
- Do not double-up on condoms—it encourages tears due to the friction between the two condoms. The tears will bring tears. And a little panic. And maybe a little surprise in nine months.
- With both male and female condoms, you must use a lubricant— inside and out—if it is not pre-lubricated. Lubrication helps prevent breakage of the condom that can be caused by friction. Oil-or petroleum-based lubricant can break down the latex, so it is best to use water-based lubricant with condoms. You do not want even the most minuscule tear—those pesky little viruses and bacteria are pretty sneaky!
- Get tested for STIs and HIV. Condoms are terrific protection— but not fool proof.
- There are many online sites that instruct how to use condoms properly, including *Planned Parenthood* and *NakedTruth Idaho*. Condom packaging typically includes instructions as well.

Female Condoms: FC2[3]

- Female condoms are inserted into the vagina before intercourse. They resemble a male condom, but are inserted similarly to a diaphragm. Lubricate!
- "Female" condom is a bit of a misnomer. Males and females can use the FC2 to protect against STIs/HIV when having anal sex. Therefore, this condom can be inserted into the vagina or anus, by any sex.
- This condom, when used correctly, is 95% effective. However most people do not use it correctly or do not use it every time they have sex therefore its effectiveness slips to 78-82%, according to the *National Institute of Health*.[4]

3   http://www.fc2femalecondom.com (2016) How to Use
4   http://www.nlm.nih.gov/medlineplus/ency/article/004002.htm (2016) Female Condoms

- FC2 is made from nitrile—which is latex-free.
- What I really love about this product is it empowers women to take charge of their sexual health in circumstances in which they have little say over their bodies.
- It can be inserted before sexual intercourse—up to 8 hours.

Dam it!

Dental dams are a thin piece of latex rubber that is used during oral-vaginal or oral-anal sex to prevent the transmission of STIs/HIV. If a person is in a pinch, non-microwaveable plastic wrap can work as well—but make sure there are no tears in it.

For more information about condoms, check out the following resources.

https://thisisl.com (L.condom)
https://www.sirrichards.com (Sir Richard)
http://sustaincondoms.com (Sustain)
http://www.trojancondoms.com (Trojan)
http://www.durex.com/pages/default.aspx (Durex)
http://www.lifestyles.com (Lifestyles)
http://www.policymic.com/articles/83255/these-3-condom-companies-want-to-help-you-save-the-world (Great article about three new condom companies)
http://www.plannedparenthood.org/health-topics/birth-control/condom (Planned Parenthood)
http://www.nakedtruth.idaho.gov (nakedtruth Idaho)

Contraception: Ladies' Choice?

What do most birth control methods have in common?? Most are forms of female contraception. The birth control pill, IUDs, implants, patches, injections are all examples of options women have. Men, however, have two option. Vasectomy, which is permanent, and the male condom. Condoms, those amazing, inexpensive little tubes of synthetic material also prevent STIs. Score one for condoms!

Does something seem a little off-balance to you? Like...maybe.... the females have to carry the burden of unintended pregnancy prevention? Well, you would be correct. But, what if the situation were reversed? Check out the hysterical *Buzz Feed Video* called *What if Buying Condoms Was Like Buying Birth Control*? (https://www.youtube.com/watch?v=9IhgwCB14To) In this video, a young man tries to obtain condoms and has to jump through the same hoops young women are required to in order to remain sexually healthy.

Yes, we can laugh at the video. It is very funny–until we realize just how unbalanced this situation is and we understand how societal norms dictate to women that they are solely responsible for their reproductive health. Yet society also makes it difficult for women to follow through with those choices. Women need to have final say in the method they use–it is their body, and they are the ones who become pregnant–not much we can do about that biological fact. But the fact remains that there are barriers for women when it comes to actually obtaining birth control.

Feeling shamed

If a young woman carries condoms in her purse or is on the pill, whispers of the woman's questionable morality might become apparent. Instead, the focus should be on her sense of responsibility.

Difficult to obtain

In order to receive a hormonal method of birth control, a young woman must visit their healthcare provider, undergo a physical exam, receive a prescription, then go to the pharmacy for pick-up. How long does that process take? At least an entire day? What if there are no health centers near her residence? What if she does not drive?

Corporations dictating what their insurance policies will cover

There is active debate simmering about who can determine the reproductive health choices of a woman; the woman? Businesses? Bosses? I don't know about you, but I just as soon make my own health choices, thank you very much.

Cost for individuals who are struggling financially

Obtaining birth control can be a difficult problem for people on limited incomes. Insurance does not always cover birth control, which surprises me since the healthcare cost of pregnancy, childbirth, and subsequently caring for a child far exceeds that of birth control.

An example of the ridiculousness women sometimes have to go through to get protection is an anecdote shared in a recent conversation with a fellow educator. He relayed an experience in which a young woman tried to purchase condoms at a pharmacy but was refused. Why? Well, she's a woman, of course. Why does *she* need a (male) condom? She walked away empty-handed, putting herself and her partner at risk for an STI and/or unintended pregnancy. That. Story. Blew. My. Mind. How fortunate that *most* places are happy to sell preventive sexual health products to consumers who care for their bodies. Thankfully, this story illustrates a rare event. However, it is eye-opening to realize what some women unnecessarily go through to keep themselves and their partners healthy.

So, what can we do? As parents, we can help raise a new generation of responsible, safe, and healthy young people by being available for conversation about reproductive health for both males and females and every gender in between.

Someday there will be a way for men to prevent pregnancy with options other than condoms or vasectomy (You want to cut WHERE????). In the meantime, teach your sons to be proactive in their partner's reproductive health. Explain to them that they can:

- Do a little research on contraception and be informed about different options.
- Discuss various methods of birth control with their partner.
- Accompany their partner to the clinic.
- Help pay for birth control.
- Remind their partner to take their birth control pill.
- Be responsible for the STI component—condoms.
- Respect their partner's choice of contraception.

Just because the ovary-owners have to worry about carrying a baby for nine months, doesn't mean the testes-owners are not accountable as well. If your child is in a same-sex relationship, this conversation should still take place. Pregnancy may not be an issue, however STIs are. Even though women are ultimately responsible for contraception, that is no excuse for it to be a woman's issue. All genders have a vested interest in contraception and should be part of the conversation.

Arm—ing Our Young Women with Protection

In September of 2014, the *American Academy of Pediatrics* (AAP) released a report written by Dr. Mary Ott and Dr. Gina Sucato and the *Committee on Adolescence* indicating that intrauterine devices (IUDs) and implants are the best method of birth control for adolescent women.[5] I was already familiar with this concept; I'd attended a conference a year or so ago in which school-based health center (SBHC) clinicians touted this as the best option for sexually-active young women. At that time, I remember thinking…what's wrong with the pill??? But I'll get back to this in a minute.

Of course, the *best* and *only* way to prevent STIs and pregnancy is abstinence. However, about half of all high school students have had sex by the time they graduate, so it is important to address topics such as contraception.

In fact, conversations about sexuality health should begin when kids are little. No, they don't need to know about intercourse at age 4. Rather, conversations about healthy relationships, learning to assert themselves, and respecting themselves and others can be woven into everyday conversation. And remember, whether you are a parent, family member, teacher…whomever…they are watching you, so model what you preach.

But I digress.

So, let's assume you and your daughter have had "the talk" (about relationships, I mean) and feel confident she understands the difference between healthy and unhealthy relationships. But now

---

5   https://www.aap.org/en-us/about-the-aap/aap-press-room/Pages/AAP-Updates-Recommendations-on-Teen-Pregnancy-Prevention.aspx (2014) AAP Updates Recommendations on Teen Pregnancy Prevention

she informs you she would like to visit the doctor for birth control. If this dialogue causes you to sweat, shake, stutter, and your eyeballs fall out, explain to her that you would like to have this conversation when you have a minute to sit and chat with her. After sipping (okay, gulping) a little wine and feel a little more relaxed and ready to listen, it is time to have an intelligent conversation with her.

Understanding the basics of birth control options for young women is the first step in engaging in this type of conversation. If you don't know which options are available, it will be difficult to sound intelligent…and we don't want them to think we don't know what we are talking about, do we???

Back to my earlier comment: So, what's wrong with the pill???

Well, nothing really. At least not when it is used correctly and consistently. And that, my friend, is the problem. With perfect use, the pill is about 99% effective. However, it is rare that the pill is used perfectly. Therefore, with typical use (yes, that's a term), the pill is about 91% effective. Not bad—unless you are the 9 in 100 who become pregnant.

You are probably wondering how a pill can be used incorrectly or inconsistently.

- It is not taken at the exact same time every day. (Setting an alarm can help.)
- Forgetting a pill here and there. (The pill must be taken at least 7 consecutive days to be effective. If you miss more than one, you must use a back-up method.)
- Taking a medication may lessen the effectiveness of the pill, therefore a back-up method should be used. (Tell your healthcare provider about all medications being taken.)
- Not refilling the prescription on time each month.

According to Dr. Ott and colleagues, the oral contraceptive pill is the most commonly used method of hormonal contraception among adolescents. The pill is also an effective way to treat other reproductive health ailments, not just for prevention of pregnancy.

But this is where the other options trump the pill. Both the IUD and the implant (which are referred to as long-acting reversible contraception—LARC), are placed into the body for between 3-12 years, depending on the device, with nary a thought! No daily reminders needed.

Wait?! What? WHERE in the body, you ask.

Contraceptive Implants:

The progestin implant, Nexplanon, is surgically inserted into the inside of the upper arm by a specially-trained healthcare provider. It's a quick procedure–about five minutes. It can be left in for up to three years.[6]

The IUD

IUDs are used commonly used world-wide; we are finally catching on to this effective method in the U.S. One type of IUD contains copper which prevents pregnancy by stopping sperm in its tracks. (They don't like copper.) This IUD can stay in the uterus about 10-12 years.

The other type of IUD contains levonorgestrel (a hormone) and also prevents sperm from making a "run for it" by causing the cervical mucus to become really thick and sticky. This type of IUD can stay in place up to 5 years, depending on the particular IUD selected.[7]

---

6   http://www.mayoclinic.org/tests-procedures/contraceptive-implant/basics/definition/prc-20015073 (2015) Contraceptive Implant

7   http://www.webmd.com/sex/birth-control/intrauterine-device-iud-for-birth-control (2015) Intrauterine Device (IUD) for Birth Control

There *is* a risk for every type of contraception. This is where a *conversation with your healthcare provider* is mandatory. Information you read here, online, in books, or discussed with friends is always helpful, but we don't know *you* or your *child*. Your physician will offer personalized care that cannot be provided anywhere else. Information given in this book and my website is merely to inform and get the conversation started. Keep in mind that by denying a sexually-active adolescent access to birth control, an unplanned pregnancy may become a reality.

Having said all this, it is important to understand that hormonal methods of contraception DO NOT protect against STIs. This is where conversation with penis-owners and vagina-owners becomes imperative. Even with the use of hormonal contraception, no matter which method works for your family member, a condom must be used in tandem to prevent the spread of STIs and HIV, unless in a monogamous relationship. In other words, sexual health responsibility does NOT lie solely with the young woman, it is a dual responsibility. After all, it does take two to tangle, does it not? Both parties should be taught to be equally responsible for the health and well-being not only of themselves, but of their partner (that's that "respect" topic mentioned earlier). And in the case of same-sex relationships in which pregnancy is not an issue, a barrier method of birth control is recommended—not to control birth, but to help both partners stay healthy.

A special thank you to Dreyer Medical Group Obstetrician and Gynecologist Dr. Caroline Mills, MD, for reviewing the original post.

May: Mother's Day and Teen Pregnancy Prevention Month
Celebrating Moms, Celebrating Choices.

May is an awesome month in my world. Spring is finally adding brilliant color and bursts of sunshine to the previously gray and dreary days of winter. The days are growing longer, which helps push my bedtime from 6 pm to 8 pm. I can finally sit outside and watch my industrious husband provide a lovely garden for my painfully short summer season.

My birthday falls in May. Though I am ever-so-thankful to keep having these annual reminders of just how old I am, I do wish we could start counting backwards. However, birthday shopping for the latest spring styles is one of my favorite pastimes; it tends to last approximately three months.

My favorite youngest daughter, Molly, also has a birthday in May. She was born two days before Mother's Day many moons ago. I have fond memories of spending that particular Mother's Day alone with an infant while the rest of the family went to brunch. I enjoyed a melted smoothie for my celebratory meal. But I digress.

Mother's Day is a momentous day in May for many women. A day to celebrate the women in our lives who have gone through the delightful agony of childbirth and adoption, only to be replaced with such joy and contentment of motherhood that they often endure the process repeatedly.

May is also Teen Pregnancy Prevention Month as put forth by *The National Campaign to Prevent Teen and Unplanned Pregnancy*. Not everyone who is a mom intended to become a mom. Or maybe they wanted to have kids one day, just not *this* day. We refer to those pregnancies as unintended pregnancies.[8] That is not to say the child subsequently brought into this great, big, beautiful world is not loved and cherished, however it can make life a little more difficult for the moms, dads, grandparents, and other family members involved in the care of the little unexpected gift.

How about some stats relating to pregnancies in the United States? You can find these and others at the *Guttmacher Institute*:[9]

- During childbearing years, about half of women will experience an unintended pregnancy
- A third of women who become unintentionally pregnant will chose to abort.
- Over the span of a woman's reproductive years, she will commit thirty years to preventing a pregnancy, and about five years of her reproductive years making, on average, two babies.
- Women who use contraceptives correctly account for only 5% of unintended pregnancies.
  According to *The National Campaign to Prevent Teen and Unplanned Pregnancy* and StayTeen.org, teen pregnancy is an issue that needs our attention.
- Twenty-five percent of women up to age 20 become pregnant.
- It costs taxpayers over $9 BILLION dollars to help out pregnant teens.
- Seventy percent of adults believe teens should have access to information about contraception and abstinence.

According to *Guttmacher Institute*, the good 'ol U.S. of A. has a teen pregnancy rate and STI infection rate higher than most other

8 http://www.cdc.gov/reproductivehealth/unintendedpregnancy/ (2015) Unintended Pregnancy Prevention
9 https://www.guttmacher.org/fact-sheet/unintended-pregnancy-united-states#8 (2016) Unintended Pregnancy in the United States

industrialized nations.[10] What can we do to ensure that women, especially women in the 15-24 year old child-bearing years, do not become pregnant unless intended?

We know abstinence is the only tried-and-true method, therefore it is an important piece of the conversation. But for argument's sake, let's refer to the statistic that about 40% of high school students have had sex by graduation.[11] And let's assume that some married couples are having sex but may not want kids right away, or ever. In both these scenarios, the problem is the same: how to prevent pregnancy at that particular time in life.

Having comprehensive sexuality health education in the classroom, whether in health class or biology class, can offer medically-accurate information that empowers individuals to make healthy choices about sex. They will understand how contraception works, how babies are made, what healthy relationships look like, and how to dialogue with partners about sex. This information benefits people whether they wait until marriage to have sex or have been sexually active throughout high school.

There are some great, medically-accurate online resources–and some really awful ones. Some young people learn about sex from pornography–and we know how accurate that information is (not!). Healthcare providers are an excellent choice when obtaining medically accurate information, however sometimes youth find it difficult to obtain information from their physicians.

---

10 https://www.guttmacher.org/news-release/2015/teen-pregnancy-rates-declined-many-countries-between-mid-1990s-and-2011 (2015) Teen Pregnancy Rates Declined In Many Countries Between The Mid-1990s and 2011

11 http://www.cdc.gov/healthyyouth/sexualbehaviors/index.htm (2016) Sexual Risk Behaviors: HIV, STD, & Teen Pregnancy Prevention

Who do teens say they are most influenced by when it comes to making decisions about sex? In other words, who should be doing most of the educating? YOU, Mom and Dad.

The National Campaign to Prevent Teen and Unplanned Pregnancy offers a tip sheet called 8 Tips for Talking to your Teen (d3np9zinex7nzb.cloudfront.net/sites/default/files/event-supporting-download/parent_tips_2016.pdf). Guide your child to *StayTeen.org* for quizzes and other information specific to young people.

On this Mother's Day weekend, when moms everywhere are basking in the indulgences of phone calls and flowers, handprints and cards, take a long look at your child. Realize that yes, they are a sexual being. Remember, they are solely responsible for your future role as grandparent. Conversations about sexuality health such as contraception, relationships, and goal-setting will empower your children to make knowledgeable and safe decisions about their health.

So for all you moms out there—birth moms, adoptive moms, foster moms, pet moms, single dads, mentors to women and girls—anyone who fulfills a nurturing and caring role in the lives of children—I wish you all the happiest of Mother's Days.

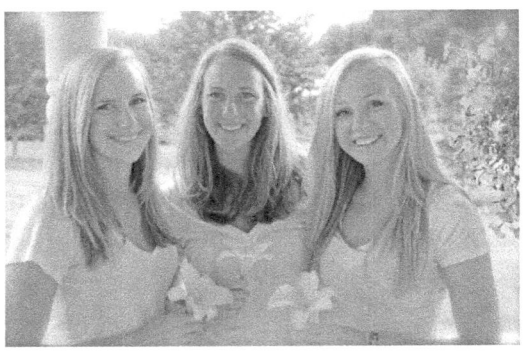

To my own daughters, you have made my life colorful and joy-filled. I cannot imagine my life without you amazing young women. *Call me*.

World Vasectomy Day

When talking about contraception, the focus is typically on the female partner within a heterosexual relationship. Likely this is because women have several options: hormonal, barrier, long acting reversible contraception (LARC), and abstinence. Rarely does the conversation transfer responsibility to the male partner–because really, there are not that many options.

Research is ongoing when it comes to contraceptive options for men. Many options cause unwanted side effects such as acne, weight gain, and mood changes.[12] Sound familiar? In the meantime, there are only a few options for men to contribute to the un-population of the world.

Certainly, condoms are typically the first and only option that comes to mind. Condoms are always a must in any sexual relationship to help prevent the spread of STIs as well as pregnancy prevention, at least until the couple is in an agreed-upon monogamous relationship. When used correctly, condoms are effective about 98% of the time. When not used correctly, that percentage drops to about 82%. When we talk about correct usage, that refers to the using a condom every single time a person has sex, using an intact and unexpired condom, and also putting it on the penis correctly and in a timely manner.

Abstinence is an option. Okay, so maybe not if we are talking about contraception at this point. Moving on…

Mutual masturbation is another method couples may choose to avoid pregnancy. It is pretty handy.

There is another option…vasectomy.

---

12 http://www.webmd.com/men/news/20160325/male-birth-control#1 (2016) Male Birth Control: More Options Soon?

Once a man (or a couple, if he is in a relationship) decides he has enough children or has chosen not to father children, he can undergo this minor surgical procedure which will permanently protect against pregnancy.

A vasectomy is an outpatient surgical procedure in which the vas deferens is snipped, clamped, or closed. This prevents jovial little sperm from moving from the testicles to the urethra to make their escape in search of the holy grail: the waiting egg. This procedure is short-a half hour or less. No, this is *not* the removal of the testes and will not affect ones manhood. Typically men can return to work in a couple of days and have sex within a week; but have a back-up method of birth control. It takes a couple of months for those little swimmers to clear out.[13]

Thinking from a woman's perspective, what a loving gesture this is! Women typically bear the burden of pregnancy prevention with years of hormones or LARC placed within their bodies. But if these methods fail, it is nine months of pregnancy, then labor and delivery, recovery, and ultimately a lifetime of care for the child. This also may affect a woman's career path. The unspoken message a man who chooses to have a vasectomy sends to his partner is, "I love you, I care about you and your health, and I respect you as a woman. Thank you for birthing our kids—it really looked like it hurt, and I'm so glad I didn't have to go through that. I can handle a little snip for our family." Okay—maybe what the male partner is really thinking is, "Geesh, these kids are expensive!" Whatever the reason, it is a terrific option when making the decision to no longer have children.

Each individual, couple, and family needs to decide what works for them when it comes to birth control options, but vasectomies are one of the few options men do have.

---

13 http://www.webmd.com/sex/birth-control/vasectomy-14387 (2015) Vasectomy

Book Review:
The Birth of the Pill by Jonathan Eig

The Birth of the Pill: How Four Crusaders Reinvented Sex and Launched a Revolution by Jonathan Eig.

Despite being an avid reader, I am not one to publicly promote books. However, I came across this informative gem of a book and was riveted. As a teacher and a nurse I feel compelled to "instruct" everyone to read this fascinating narrative that altered the course of humankind.

Let me ask you something. When you consider your birth control choices and access to it, what is the first thing that comes to your mind? Prescriptions? Cost? Ease-of-use? Thank-God-I-Only-Had-Two-Children? If you are like me, the ability to control our personal birth rate is something I never truly appreciated. I wanted three kids. I had three kids. Not 6. Not 10. And it was a decision between my husband and myself. Not just my husband. Not the government. Not my doctor. Not our religious leaders. Kind of a no-brainer. Couples make a choice that is best for their family. (Wellllll…there *are* those occasional "oops.")

It never dawned on me just how incredibly fortunate Western society is to have these options when just a mere 50 years ago (Yes! My lifetime!) women were literally begging for help, desperate to control their personal birth rates.

How about an example many mothers can relate to?

(Cue the sound of happy, chirping birds…) You awake on a beautiful, sunny morning and gaze lovingly into your well-behaved, compliant,

perfectly attired children. You reflect on the previous romantic evening with your life partner in which the love-making was earth-shattering and mutually satisfying. You prepare to go off to work where you are appreciated and adequately paid. Or maybe you chose to be a stay-at-home mother…which means you will soon be off and running to some committee meeting or another. Life is good.

Okay. Maybe that is fantasy world. But consider what reality was a mere 50-60 years ago:

(Cue the sound of roosters crowing…) You awake on a lovely, sunny morning and your eyes glaze over the 5 to 10 children standing at your feet looking for something to eat for breakfast. You are exhausted because, even though you love your husband, you realize the dutiful quickie last night will likely result in another baby—one you are not physically, mentally, or emotionally prepared to care for. A worried, sleepless night followed. The weariness is taking its toll. You are unsure if all your children are present and accounted for; "how many rug-rats do I have now?" you ponder. No matter. If they are hungry they will show up. You pick up a bowl and start kneading the dough for today's bread and begin the routine of caring for your brood. You love them, but the exhaustion is getting the better of you. If only there was a way to limit the number of children born to you. Some magic pill. You know someone that performs abortions…should you try that? So many women die when they try to abort, yet the thought of another child to care for is disheartening and overwhelming. Desperate times, desperate measures.

This is a reality of women's history that is not taught in our schools. However, The Birth of the Pill by Jonathan Eig documents the journey of four innovative individuals with a passion to improve the lives of all humanity, not only women.

Margaret Sanger: Famous for founding *Planned Parenthood*, Sanger understood that sex could be fun for women as well as men—not just a baby-making activity. She wanted women to have the ability to control their fertility, and therefore of their lives. Can you imagine that it was not considered "OK" for women to enjoy sex? Aye Aye Aye. Thank you, Margaret!

Katharine McCormick: An MIT graduate (unheard of back in 1920's), the wealthy McCormick financed the research for the pill. She felt there was no point in championing for women's rights and higher education until women had reproductive freedom. Without the ability to prevent unwanted pregnancies, women would never be free to live their authentic lives. Sadly, McCormick's desire to have The Pill available for women in impoverished and developing countries was never realized in her lifetime—and has yet to be realized in ours. Re-read that second scenario…it is a reality for many women around the world.

Gregory Pincus: A brilliant visionary and scientist who believed anything was possible when it came to reproductive health—and was willing to do whatever it took to make it happen.

John Rock: A Catholic gynecologist who felt this natural method of birth control would be a perfect fit with the church's teachings. Rock and Pincus set out on a journey of research and compassion that would change the world.

Sanger and McCormick understood the physical, mental, and social implications this little innovative pill would have on women, children, families, communities worldwide. Combining their passion and talent they were a force to be reckoned with. Because this was the first drug developed for something other than a treatment for disease or illness, their research methods and the evidence they offered to back up their results were quite sketchy; their methods would not be respected in this day and age. Thank goodness they were rebels in their field!

To truly understand and appreciate our modern-day birth control options, digging into the history about the perseverance of these four random visionaries who pursued their passion and entwined their talents is a must. I predict this will be a movie. Yes. It is that entertaining. (I see the plucky Jennifer Lawrence playing a young Margaret Sanger...Just sayin'.)

"Mom, We're Pregnant." Moving Forward When Your World is Rocked

I was fortunate enough to sit next to a very interesting and inspiring woman on the plane the other day. Her most recent work involves caring for and counseling people who have HIV/AIDS. Naturally, our conversations revolved around "how to change the world." But since neither of us has any political aspirations, we agreed that we can change our little corners of the world by having conversations with others that may impact their lives in a positive way. And what can I say? I like to talk about sex!

As our flight was descending, she requested I address one discussion in particular: The importance of parents in supporting their children when life hits them hard.

Imagine this scenario...

It is a lovely autumn afternoon. You are relaxing while reading the latest sexy romance novel tucked inside a recent National Geographic (no worries, I won't tell), when your son approaches you with a very serious look on his face. So many things go through your mind; he crashed the car, he flunked a test, he flunked out of school (!), he doesn't want to go to Grandma's tonight...Whatever it is, it can't be THAT bad. Whatever it is, it will be resolved as soon as he spills.

But wait. What was that? What did he say? You don't think you heard this correctly. His girlfriend is what? Pregnant? What??!! Since when??!! They are only 16 years old! They CAN'T be sexually active yet...can they?

Your response is to...

A. *Start screaming and yelling "What were you thinking????"*
B. *Start sobbing uncontrollably.*
C. *Look at him and say, "Okay, joke's up."*
D. *Don't say anything you will regret, get your thoughts together, give him a hug, and tell him you need a minute. Walk away, grab the wine and someone to talk to.*

Well, we all know the obvious answer is D (with or without the wine, however). But if you reflexively chose A, B, or C, I won't judge. I understand it is shocking, scary, and maybe dream-shattering–at least in that moment.

So, how do you move forward? We have all made mistakes. Some mistakes are quite trivial, and others rather shocking, scary, and dream-shattering. And if you haven't, Ms or Mr. Perfect, I'm sure you know someone who has. Think about how you or someone you know (wink) has worked through seemingly insurmountable problems. I'm betting they gained wisdom and courage to help them grapple with future distressing predicaments. That's how life works.

You have to make a choice. You can dwell on the problem ("Why me? What will the neighbors think? How could they have done this? I'm so embarrassed. Their life is overrrrrrr!") Or, you can be a part of the solution by continuing to move forward with the situation at hand.

After you've calmed yourself down, take your son by the hand. Tell him you love him. Tell him you will get through this together. This sounds pretty fairy-tale. I get it. I also know that there will be "discussions" of "disappointment". However, keep it in check–be kind and acknowledge this probably was not on his immediate bucket list either. Put yourself in his (shaking) shoes.

Let me help you reframe your thoughts. Let's back away from the idea that certain life situations are "problems" and appreciate that they are, well…"certain life situations." A friend once told me: "Don't admire the problem, work towards the solution."

In the past, I've written about helping your child make good choices based on their values and purpose in life. I suggested asking them a few questions, two of which are:

- *Where do you see yourself in 5 (or 10) years?*
- *How do you see yourself achieving this goal/dream?*

Well, now I want you to ask yourself these questions:

- *What kind of relationship do you hope to have with your child 5 (or 10) years from now?*
- *How do you see yourself building that relationship?*

So, you tell me. With those four choices up there, which one makes the most sense? Freaking out? Or working together to come up with a plan?

Yeah. I thought so.

"In any moment of decision, the best thing you can do is the right thing. The worst thing you can do is nothing." Theodore Roosevelt

Planning for Parenthood

Despite the prevalence of health care clinics in nearly every community, whether it be within a hospital, school, private medical clinic, or even in the local grocery store, many people are unable to access or afford medical care when needed. This may be due to lack of insurance, inability to afford care, or the individual may not be aware of community medical resources.

However, one clinic is known throughout the land. It has withstood the test of time, having first formed 101 years ago in 1916.[14] The formidable and determined Margaret Sanger understood the need for women to have more autonomy in their lives, and the first step was to allow women to plan their parenthood. Thank goodness, right?! I have three kids and that was more than enough for me. I cannot imagine how my life would have been without the option to choose the size of my family. Those nights out with girlfriends, enjoying a glass of wine, discussing political issues—or not—would not be an option.

Planned Parenthood is one of the most recognized and respected medical providers for women—and men—in the world.

Five million people are provided health education and healthcare through Planned Parenthood's services around the globe.

Services include annual exams for women, cancer screenings, vasectomies, and STI testing.[15,16]

---

14 https://www.plannedparenthood.org/planned-parenthood-heartland/who-we-are/history (2016) History of Planned Parenthood of the Heartland.

15 https://www.plannedparenthoodaction.org/issues/health-care-equity/title-x (2016) Title X: America's Family Planning Program

16 http://www.cnn.com/2015/08/04/health/planned-parenthood-by-the-numbers/ (2015) Planned Parenthood: Fast facts and revealing numbers.

42% of Planned Parenthood's services are STI screenings.

80% of Planned Parenthood's patients want to prevent a pregnancy.[17]

Merely 3% of Planned Parenthood's services are abortion procedures.

60 million people visit Planned Parenthood's website a year.[18] Their website offers medically-accurate reproductive health information to allow individuals to make informed decisions regarding their reproductive health. The information is current and easy to understand. There are videos, handouts, visuals, and interesting articles for young people, parents and professionals. No matter the question, there is an answer there.

In 1970 Title X was passed that allows federal funding for organizations such as Planned Parenthood and other family planning centers to provide education, health care services, research, and pregnancy prevention to low-income individuals. According to Planned Parenthood, "Title X also saves taxpayers money. For every dollar invested in publicly funded family planning programs, the government saves $7.09 in Medicaid-related costs."[19] Not only does Planned Parenthood provide individuals with excellent healthcare, birth control, and education among many other services, it also helps the government save money, not to mention families.

I am proud to say that many, many moons ago I was a volunteer birth control educator at Planned Parenthood. I saw women of all ages seeking help–some as young as 12. Thank goodness they had a safe place to go for quality care. Birth control, education,

17 http://www.cnn.com/2015/08/04/health/planned-parenthood-by-the-numbers/
     (2015) Planned Parenthood: Fast facts and revealing numbers.
18 https://www.plannedparenthood.org/files/7214/6833/9709/20160711_FS_
     PPNumbers_d1.pdf (2016) By the Numbers
19 https://www.plannedparenthoodaction.org/issues/health-care-equity/title-x
     (2016) Title X: America's Family Planning Program

and check-ups were happily provided despite a person's ability to pay. The quality of the organization impressed me; my short time at Planned Parenthood set me on the path that continues to inspire me. It ignited a passion in me that has been simmering over the last three decades–to offer emerging adults comprehensive reproductive education and healthcare to help prevent unwanted pregnancies. If we teach about birth control, abortion can be greatly reduced. Planned Parenthood sets out to do exactly as its name states: to plan parenthood.

Kim T. Cook, RN CHES

"Is sex safe?" Male, 10th grade

"Can you tell if someone has an STD?" Male, 11th grade

"Can you get STDs from oral sex?" Male, 11th grade

"Can all types of sex lead to STDs?" Male, 11th grade

SEXUALLY TRANSMITTED INFECTIONS (STIs):

hazardous conditions ahead

VD-STD-STI...What Does It All Mean??

Many of us are familiar with the term "STD", but "STI" and "VD" may not be as familiar to you.

Long ago in a faraway land...well, really up until the 1990's, VD (venereal disease) was the term typically used when discussing sexually transmitted infections and disease. Since that time, STD (sexually transmitted disease) became the preferred terminology of healthcare providers.

In the last few years, to add to everyone's confusion, a new term came on board—STI—which stands for sexually transmitted infection. Why oh why must we learn yet another term??

Well, chances are you will not hear the term VD very often anymore. In fact, I heard it just the other day, and it caught me off-guard—that is the only reason I am even addressing it.

Having said that, I would like you to be familiar with the difference in the terms STI and STD—after all, you DO want to be the really cool adult in the room who actually *knows* the difference, right?

An STI—"I" meaning *infection*—means that a person can have a sexually transmitted virus, bacteria, or parasite that may or may not show symptoms. In other words, they may have an infection and not even realize it. That is a problem, of course, when considering their future partners who will then be unknowingly exposed. Yikes.

An STD—"D" meaning *disease*—means that a person is showing symptoms of the viral, bacterial, or parasitic infection and should get help...well, *yesterday!*

Also, there is another reason to use the term STI—it is just a little bit more "gentle." After all, everyone gets some sort of infection at some point in time—sinus, bladder, toe—and no one really thinks it is super embarrassing. However, a disease can sound somewhat dreadful, and people might be embarrassed to talk about it or get help from a healthcare provider. Healthcare providers want patients to feel comfortable getting proper medical care, of course! After all, these infections are highly contagious—we don't really want to re-gift this little surprise.

So there you have it. In 300 words, you have learned the difference between STI and STD. Most people use these terms interchangeably. It is not really a big deal if you do. I personally prefer using STI as a general rule, so that is how I will address these infections/diseases.

_____

Understanding the Basics of Sexually Transmitted Infections

Let's walk down the path to understanding the most common types of STIs. We have heard a lot about HPV lately, with the somewhat recent introduction of HPV vaccines for our kids. HIV/AIDS is frequently in the news as well. And then there are the "usual" STI's: herpes, gonorrhea, chlamydia. And how about crabs???

Obviously, there are many infections we need to be aware of. But not all infections are created equal! We can break down these infections into three basic categories: bacterial, viral, and parasitic. These categories can help us understand the "how" and "why" of treatment, as there is no "cure-all" for STI's.

Bacterial: Bacteria are single-celled microorganisms that can live just about anywhere, inside or outside the body. Simply put, they cause infection by moving from one reservoir (a place they are hanging out, like your body) to another reservoir (like someone else's body). Not all bacteria are bad–we need some to keep us healthy, like in our intestines. But right now, we're talking about sexually transmitted bacterial infections. The old school classics like chlamydia, gonorrhea, and syphilis can now be cured with antibiotics, which will significantly decrease the chance of any long-term negative health effect due to the infection, if caught early enough. Unfortunately, individuals may have a bacterial STI and not have any symptoms for a while, which is why we are encouraged to get tested regularly if sexually active.

Viral: Viruses are tricky because they like to live *in* our cells; they take advantage of their new home and reproduce themselves within the cell. The cell will burst open, and the newly formed viruses then invade other nearby cells, repeating the process. This can, and usually will, cause disease and even cancer. The common cold is an example of a viral infection. Examples of sexually transmitted viruses are human papillomavirus (HPV), herpes, human immunodeficiency virus (HIV), Hepatitis B, Hepatitis C, and more recently, the Zika virus. These cannot be cured with antibiotics. However, depending on the virus, there are treatments available to help with the symptoms, the progress of the disease, and even the prevention of disease. As with bacterial STI's, viral STI's may not present with any signs or symptoms at first. Another reason to get tested regularly.

Parasitic: Parasites are organisms that live on another organism. And by living on it, I mean dining and relaxing on their host organism. Ticks are one example of a type of parasite, as are intestinal worms. However, sexually transmitted parasites include pubic lice (crabs) and trichomoniaisis. These infections are treatable.

As you can tell, there are lots of ways a person can become infected with an STI. Sometimes you can treat it, sometimes you can't. However, there are ways to prevent them. My personal philosophy is to prevent, prevent, prevent.

Bacterial Vaginosis (BV)

Overview:

- An imbalance of the bacteria of the vagina.
- It is the most common vaginal infection in women.
- VB should not be confused with a yeast infection; yeast infections are caused by an imbalance of the yeast fungus.[1] (Yeast and bacteria are normally present in the vagina.)

Causes:

- Anyone can get it–*whether or not they are sexually active.* If a vagina-owner is diagnosed with BV, it does not necessarily mean they were infected by engaging in sexual activity.
- It can be spread with female-to-female sexual activity.

Symptoms and Effects:

- Often silent.
- It can be characterized by a fishy odor, burning when urinating, itching around the vagina, and/or discharge.
- It increases the chance of contracting another STI.
- If pregnant, be sure to get treated. It can cause premature delivery or low birth weight.
- Can cause PID if untreated.

Treatment:

- BV is treated with antibiotics. Take the full prescribed dose!

---

1   https://www.cdc.gov/fungal/diseases/candidiasis/genital (2014) Genital / vulvovaginal candidiasis (VVC)

- Men do not need to be treated.
- As always, talk to a doc (or other healthcare provider) if you have any concerns.

Prevention:

- Abstinence.
- Limit the number of sexual partners.
- Avoid douching.

The CDC was the primary source for this information: http://www.cdc.gov/STD/bv/STDFact-Bacterial-Vaginosis.htm (2016) Bacterial Vaginosis (BV)

Please remember–this information is NOT intended to be used to self-diagnose or replace any medical advice your healthcare provider will give you. It is only to inform and educate. Please see your healthcare provider if you have any questions, problems, symptoms, issues, and concerns regarding your sexual health.

Chlamydia

What is it?

- It is caused by the bacterium *Chlamydia trachomatis*.
- The most common bacterial STI. 1 in 15 (sexually active) females 14-19 have it according to the CDC.
- Individuals 25 and under are more likely to contract this, and women have an even higher chance of getting it.
- Non-hispanic blacks are also at higher risk.
- HIV-infected individuals have an increased risk of getting chlamydia.

Causes:

- This STI is spread by oral, anal, or vaginal sexual activity.

Symptoms and Effects:

- It's silent. In other words, people usually don't realize they have it because there usually are no symptoms.
- Females may feel burning when urinating and notice a discharge from their vagina. There may be abdominal pain.
- Guys may also have burning with urination. They may have testicular pain.
- Long-term consequences of untreated chlamydia include:
  In women: Pelvic Inflammatory Disease (PID). This occurs when the bacteria attacks the female reproductive system. The end result can be infertility and ectopic pregnancy. Repeated chlamydia infections can make permanent consequences more likely. (This is why it is so important for women to get tested.)
  In newborns: It can cause pre-term birth or eye infections.
  In guys: (Very rare) Infection that could cause sterility.

Treatment:

- Because it is a bacterial Infection it can be treated and cured with antibiotics. However, a person can get this infection repeatedly. In fact, they often do. Don't have sex for 7 days after the start of your antibiotics…give the medication a little time to kick in and kick some bacterial butt.
- All of the sexual partners the individual has had in the last 2 months must be notified.
- Re-test 3 months after treatment to make sure all is well.

Prevention:

- Abstinence.
- Use a latex condom or female condom–and use it correctly to be fully effective.
- Be monogamous. Both partners!
- Get tested. Diagnosis is made with a urine screen or swab (endocervical, anal, urethral, or vaginal).
  Sexually active woman, 25-years-old or younger, should be tested annually. (Oral, vaginal, anal–doesn't matter what kind of sex…)
  If a woman is older than 25, and has had a new sexual partner(s), get tested annually.
  If a guy is having anal sex with another guy, they are at risk. So get tested annually.
  If you are pregnant, get tested (it can affect the baby).
  If your partner has just been diagnosed, get tested.
  Routine screening for sexually active guys isn't generally recommended, but it is for sexually active young women.
  In other words, get tested if for any reason at all you feel you might be at risk.
  The CDC was the primary source for this information: http://www.cdc.gov/std/chlamydia/stdfact-chlamydia. htm (2016) Chlamydia-CDC Fact Sheet

For more information:

http://www.cdc.gov/std/chlamydia/chlam-fact-sheet-press-dec-2012.pdf

http://www.plannedparenthood.org/health-topics/stds-hiv-safer-sex/chlamydia-4266.htm

http://kidshealth.org/parent/infections/std/chlamydia.html#

Please remember–this information is NOT intended to be used to self-diagnose or replace any medical advice your healthcare provider will give you. It is only to inform and educate. Please see your healthcare provider if you have any questions, problems, symptoms, issues, and concerns regarding your sexual health.

Gonorrhea

Overview:

- Gonorrhea is a sexually transmitted infection caused by the bacterium *Neisseria gonorrhoeae*.
- Very common. Just over 800,000 people are diagnosed each year.
- This bacterium really likes warm moist environments like the urethra, throat, mouth, anus, and eyes in both males and females, and the reproductive tract of females.
- Individuals aged 15-24 are infected with it more frequently than other age groups.
- Women are infected more frequently than men.
- Because it is a bacterial infection, it can be treated and cured with antibiotics. However, a person can be repeatedly infected. In fact, they often are.

Causes

- This disease is spread by sexual contact and during childbirth.

Symptoms and Effects:

- Symptoms may be silent, so the individual may not be aware they are infected.
- Chlamydia is often diagnosed along with gonorrhea.
- Gals: May feel pain when urinating and notice a discharge or bleeding from their vagina. Sometimes it is misdiagnosed as a bladder infection.
- Guys: May have a discharge from their penis, pain when urinating, and/or scrotal pain up to two weeks after exposure.

- Long-term consequences of untreated gonorrhea include:
  In women: Pelvic Inflammatory Disease (PID). This occurs when the bacteria attacks the female reproductive system. The end result can be infertility and ectopic pregnancy. Repeated gonorrhea infections can make permanent consequences more likely.
  In newborns: blindness, infection
  In guys: (very rare) infection that could cause sterility

Treatment:

- Antibiotics. Sadly, antibiotics previously used to treat this are no longer as effective, therefore it is becoming difficult to treat. This is called anti-microbial resistance. This is also why healthcare providers tell people to take *all of* the prescribed antibiotics (no matter what the ailment)–a person mustn't stop just because they feel better. Treatment for gonorrhea typically consists of two medications rather than just one (because of this resistance).
- Do not have sex until all medication has been taken–it's no fun to share this!
- Tell all sexual partners they've been with in the last two months (oral, vaginal, anal).
- Get re-tested if symptoms persist.
- Take all of the prescribed meds, even if they are feeling better! (Have I mentioned this before?)

Prevention:

- Well, abstain; it is the only guaranteed way a person will not become pregnant or get an STI.
- Use latex male condoms or female condoms–and use them correctly to be fully effective.
- Be monogamous–both partners!

- Get tested for STIs:
- Before initiating sex with a new partner; any kind of sex–oral, anal, or vaginal.
- Their partner was recently diagnosed with it–or any other STI for that matter.
- They notice any unusual symptoms "down under" such as a discharge, discomfort, or rash.
- If pregnant, get tested. (It can seriously affect the baby.)
- In other words, get tested if for any reason at all you feel you might be at risk.
- Talk to the doc if you are sexually active. This includes oral, anal, or vaginal sex.

The CDC was the primary source for this information: http://www.cdc.gov/std/gonorrhea/stdfact-gonorrhea-detailed.htm (2016) Gonorrhea-CDC Fact Sheet (Detailed Version)

For more information:

- http://www.cdc.gov/std/gonorrhea/gon-fact-sheet-june-2012.pdf
- http://kidshealth.org/teen/sexual_health/stds/std_gonorrhea.html
- http://www.plannedparenthood.org/health-topics/stds-hiv-safer-sex/gonorrhea-4269.htm

Please remember–this information is not intended to be used to self-diagnose or replace any medical advice your healthcare provider will give you. It is only to inform and educate. Please see your healthcare provider if you have any questions, problems, symptoms, issues, and concerns regarding your sexual health.

No Need to Go Crazy: Understanding Syphilis

Overview:

- Syphilis is an STI caused by the bacterium *Treponema pallidum*
- About 74,000 people were diagnosed in 2015, the highest rates in men 20-29 years old.
- In 2015, almost 82% of all first and second stage syphilis had been reported in MSM (*m*en who have *s*ex with *m*en).
- It is typically found in racial and ethnic minorities.
- Excluding the MSM population, black males have the highest rate of primary and secondary syphilis.
- **Congenital syphilis** (syphilis passed on to a newborn at birth) has risen in the past couple years from 162 to 487 cases in 2015. These numbers were higher among black and Hispanic infants.

Causes:

- A chancre, or sore, carries the bacteria. Contact through that sore via oral, anal, or vaginal sex spreads the disease.
- A mother can pass syphilis on her to newborn child during childbirth, known as congenital syphilis.

Symptoms and Effects:

- Symptoms look like a lot of other diseases and tend to go away on their own, therefore people may not get tested. However, the bacteria continue to lurk in the body.
- Because it is a bacterial infection, it can be treated, especially during the first and second stages of the disease.

- Pregnant women should be tested for syphilis and again after delivery. Babies born to women with untreated syphilis may have one of many different and very serious health problems
- There are four stages of syphilis with distinct signs and symptoms in each stage.

Primary Stage

- It takes about 21 days to 3 months to show the first symptoms.
- One or more chancres, or sores, will develop. Typically, they are seen in the rectum, on the vagina, anus, or penis.
- They can also be found on the lips and mouth.
- The chancres don't hurt, and only last about 3-6 weeks before they just disappear.
- Chancres may not be easy to see.
- However, these sores cause the spread of the disease during sexual activity.
- Symptoms may be gone…but not forgotten…because if it is not treated by simple antibiotics, it moves on to ….

Secondary Stage

- A red or brownish rash may appear on the palms of the hands or skin…or it may not even be visible. Other rashes may appear as well but might look very similar to other illnesses.
- The person may also have symptoms a lot like the flu: fever, muscle aches, sore throat, headaches, and fatigue, for example.
- A person may also find sores showing up on their mucous membranes such as the mouth, vagina, or anus.
- These symptoms will disappear after a while, however, the disease is still lurking….

- Symptoms may be gone…but not forgotten…because if it is not treated with simple antibiotics, it moves on to...

The Third Stage: The Latent Stage

- The person is infected and does not know it–or believes they are no longer ill–because there are no obvious signs or symptoms–it is latent–just sort of hanging around, quietly doing damage.
- Depending on when a person was infected, they may have "early" or "late" latent syphilis.
- Symptoms may be gone…but not forgotten…because if it's not treated with simple antibiotics, it moves on to…

The Late Stages

- Syphilis can appear as long as two decades after being infected in about 15% of untreated individuals.
- Damage occurs to internal organs, such as the brain, eyes, liver, heart, etc.
- With that damage, the individual may experience numbness, blindness, paralysis, dementia or even death.
  Need I say more?

Treatment:

Antibiotics will rid the body of the disease. However, persons can become reinfected.

Prevention:

- Abstain. It is the only guaranteed method to prevent STIs or pregnancy.
- Get tested. Testing is simple: a blood test or a fluid sample from the chancre.

- Monogamous relationship–both of you. But you must be tested before your first sexual encounter.
- If your partner has tested positive for syphilis, then you should be tested as well.
- Even if you have been treated for it once before, you can get it again.
- *Proper* and *consistent* use of latex condoms and/or dental dams. (Remember, birth control pills, IUDs, and implants are to decrease your risk of pregnancy. They do nothing to prevent STIs.)

BE SAFE. BE TESTED. BE TREATED.

The CDC was the primary source for this information: http://www.cdc.gov/std/syphilis/stdfact-syphilis.htm (2016) Syphilis-CDC Fact Sheet

Please remember–this information is NOT intended to be used to self-diagnose or replace any medical advice your healthcare provider will give you. It is only to inform and educate. Please see your healthcare provider if you any questions, problems, symptoms, issues, and concerns regarding your sexual health.

Herpes

Did you know innocent-looking cold sores are actually a form of herpes?

Herpes simplex 1, or HSV-1, is the virus that causes cold sores visible around the lips and in the mouth.[2] Sharing beverages, sharing silverware or cups, kissing, etc. enhances the spread of the virus, often in childhood.

Herpes simplex 2, or HSV-2, is the virus that causes blisters around the genitalia and rectum.[3] Typically when someone uses the word 'herpes' this is the infection to which they are referring. This virus is spread primarily by oral, anal, or vaginal sexual encounters.

Herpes is a viral infection–it cannot be cured. However there are medications to lesson symptoms and help prevent breakouts. Antibiotics do not work for this viral infection. Both strains of the herpes virus cause oral and genital herpes.

Genital herpes often shows no symptoms or may look nondescript–like a little pimple–so the owner of this disease does not realize they are infected and may unknowingly share it with their partner. Signs or symptoms of genital herpes may include a general sense of not feeling well and one or more fluid-filled blisters and/or sores around the infected area (including the mouth as well as the vagina, penis, and rectum). The fluid inside the blisters is loaded with the virus. Hand-washing is a must. Avoid touching other parts of the body–the virus is not too particular where it resides; even the eyes. Typically after the first year symptoms occur less frequently, but the virus will continue to inhabit the infected person's body. In other

---

2   http://kidshealth.org/en/teens/cold-sores.html# Cold Sores (HSV-1)
3   http://www.webmc.com/genital-herpes/guide/what-is-it#1 (1999) Genital Herpes

words, the virus can still be shared amongst lovers even as the symptoms lessen over time.

The only way to prevent infection is to abstain. In fact, that is the only way to ever prevent any STI or pregnancy. Since most humans eventually have sex, this is not always practical advice. Using a condom properly can *help* prevent infection, but because any skin contact can transfer the virus, it is not super effective against this particular STI. Just the same, use a condom. Please.

If you or your partner have an STI, get tested for herpes as well. If you have the slightest question about having contracted herpes, get tested. If you are entering into a new intimate relationship, you and your partner should be tested for STI's, including herpes. If you or your partner has a herpes outbreak, abstain from sex until the symptoms are gone, which can take up to a month. See your healthcare provider for care and guidance.

It is important to talk to your partner about your sexual health, especially when it comes to sexually transmitted infections. It is not always an easy conversation, but in a committed, loving relationship it will help build intimacy.

For more information, go to the CDC website: Genital Herpes–STD Fact Sheet.[4]

---

4   http://www.cdc.gov/std/herpes/stdfact-herpes.htm (2016) Genital Herpes - STD Fact Sheet

Reduce the Risk: HPV

We know that human papillomavirus (HPV) is a virus that has about 40 sexually transmitted strains.[5] Some strains cause more problems than others, the worst being genital warts and cancer, especially cervical cancer. Our body can get rid of some strains without a hitch, and some it can't. Unfortunately, we don't know which kind of HPV we might come into contact with, and we don't know which strain(s) our body will be able to fight off.

So, here's the deal. These are the suggestions the medical community gives to help reduce the risk of HPV and the diseases it can cause.

Remain abstinent. If a person isn't having sex (oral, anal, vaginal–it's all sex), they cannot get an STI. End of story. However, at the point in life they choose to begin a sexual relationship they will need to have a sexual health plan.

Stay in a monogamous relationship. The less people an individual has sex with, the less chance they have of becoming infected.

Use a condom. A person and their partner may not actually *know* if they have HPV–there may be no symptoms. HPV is spread by being in contact with a partner's skin, especially down in the nether-regions. If a condom is used–male or female condom–before *any* skin contact, it can help decrease the odds of (but NOT necessarily prevent) getting HPV and the diseases that come with it, like genital warts and cervical cancer. Just make sure the condom is used correctly.

---

5   http://www.webmd.com/sexual-conditions/hpv-genital-warts/hpv-virus-information-about-human-papillomavirus#1 (2015) Information About the Human Papillomavirus (HPV)

Get a Pap test. People who happen to have a cervix should continue to get this screening for cervical cancer. Talk to a healthcare provider for information.

Be sure your child gets the cancer vaccine. Oh, I mean the HPV vaccine. The medical community is being encouraged to refer to this preventative measure as a cancer vaccine because that is precisely what we are trying to prevent–*cancer*! Oral. Anal. Penile. Vulvar. Throat. Cervical. According to *The National Cancer Institute*, "HPV infection accounts for about 5% of all cancers worldwide."[6] As an extra bonus, this vaccine can prevent genital warts as well. This vaccine is "extremely effective" in preventing infections due to HPV (CDC).[7]

This vaccine is approved for both genders. It is recommended it be given before a person is sexually active–which makes sense since you can contract HPV the first time you have sex. The really smart people that research this stuff all the time say age 11-ish is a good time to begin, generally speaking. It's a series of two or three shots–so don't forget to get them all!![8] Besides abstinence, it really is the best *prevention* we have.

Gardasil and Cervarix

There are two vaccines currently available. Gardasil 9 is for both sexes. It protects against 9 strains of HPV, which are known to cause warts and the different cancers discussed earlier, especially cervical cancer. Cervarix is given to females and protects against 2 strains of HPV that can cause cervical cancer. Both are very effective.

---

6 https://www.cancer.gov/about-cancer/causes-prevention/risk/infectious-agents/hpv-fact-sheet (2015) HPV and cancer

7 http://www.cdc.gov/vaccines/vpd/hpv/index.html (2016)Human Papillomavirus (HPV) Vaccination & Cancer Prevention

8 http://www.cdc.gov/media/releases/2016/p1020-hpv-shots.html (2016) CDC recommends only two HPV shots for younger adolescents

Parent Concerns

I know a lot of parents have concerns about this vaccine, which as a parent/caregiver, you *should* question what is going into your child's body. Kudos to you! Let me run down some of your concerns and what the studies have shown.

• Why so young??

Because it's likely they haven't had sex yet. No point in giving a vaccine to someone after they have the virus, right?

• If they have this vaccine, the kids will think it's *party time* and will actively go out and have sex.

Um. No. Really? I don't even think my kids knew what this "shot" was for. You go to the doctor and you get a shot. Do they always ask you the details of their vaccines? I didn't think so. Plus, the CDC says research was done on this, and it turns out it does not effect when adolescents start having sex. In fact, I think this would be an awesome opportunity to talk about sex and your values, morals, thoughts with your child. Research has shown that parent conversation has a huge impact on kids!

• My child isn't having sex. They won't be exposed to HPV.

Read my blurb about abstinence, up above.

• Side effects!!!! My child could die if they have the vaccine!

I can tell you from personal experience the only side-effect my girls experienced was soreness at the site of injection. As of now, research has shown there are "no long-term side effects and no serious safety concerns have been identified."[9] That is a direct quote from the CDC. A little mild

---

9   http://www.cdc.gov/hpv/parents/questions-answers.html (2016) HPV Questions and answers

discomfort from a vaccine is nothing compared to dealing with genital warts or cancer.

Having said that, as a responsible parent, have a conversation with your healthcare provider about allergies your child may have with certain ingredients in the medication. Also, discuss the rare immediate side effects reported, such as fever, nausea, headache, and dizziness.

Want to know more? The following web addresses can provide more information.

http://www.cervarix.ca
http://www.gardasil.com
vaccine.chip.edu
http://kidshealth.org/teen/sexual_health/stds/std_warts. html#cat20017
http://www.cdc.gov/vaccines/vpd-vac/hpv/default.htm
http://www.cancer.gov/cancertopics/factsheet/Risk/HPV
http://www.cancer.gov/cancertopics/factsheet/prevention/HPV-vaccine
https://www.plannedparenthood.org/parents/talking-to-kids-about-sex-and-sexuality

Please remember–this information is not intended to be used to self-diagnose or replace any medical advice your healthcare provider will give you. It is only to inform and educate. Please see your healthcare provider if you have any questions, problems, symptoms, issues, and concerns regarding your sexual health.

HPV Vaccine:
Know the Facts, Make the Choice

What is Human Papillomavirus?

Let me begin by emphasizing that HPV is not the same virus as HIV. The abbreviations look very similar. However, HIV is human immunodeficiency virus, the virus that may develop into AIDS.

Human papilloma virus, or HPV, on the other hand, is a virus that is also spread through sexual contact, but not necessarily sexual intercourse.[10] The virus is happy with a little skin contact. Therefore, it is very easily spread, even when using a condom. In fact, 80% of all people have been infected with this virus at some point.[11] If you have had sex, you probably have had HPV at some point. Yes, you likely have had a sexually transmitted infection (STI) and did not even know it–it typically does not present any symptoms.

There are over 150 types of HPV, 40 of which are sexually transmitted.[12] Fortunately for most people, our body's immune system is able to deal with HPV; after about 6 months to a couple of years the body naturally rids itself of the virus.

However, there are certain strains that have been identified as troublemakers for some people. These particular strains may cause cervical cancer, anal cancer, penile cancer, vulvar cancer, vaginal cancer and a variety of oral cancers (mouth, throat). Other strains may cause genital warts.

---

10 http://www.cdc.gov/hpv (2016) Human Papillomavirus (HPV)

11 http://www.hpv.com.au (2016) Understanding HPV

12 http://www.cdc.gov/hpv/parents/whatishpv.html (2015) What is HPV?

Please note that different strains cause different infections: Strains that cause cancer do not typically cause warts, and vice-versa.

Currently, there is no way to predict whether:

- a daughter is going to be one of the 120,000 women diagnosed with cervical cancer each year.[13]
- a child will be one of the growing number of individuals diagnosed with other cancers such as penile, oral, or anal. Currently the number is almost 35,000 a year.[14]
- a child will be one of 355,000 people diagnosed each year with genital warts.
- a child will ever have any diseases caused by HPV infection.

Vaccination

One mother wrote and asked:

"As a mom to a 9-year-old girl, the topic of HPV vaccines will be quickly approaching my radar. I don't necessarily understand the vaccine itself. Does it completely prevent the virus? Are boosters required down the road if my daughter gets the initial vaccine?"

Excellent question, and one that every parent of a youngster should be evaluating. The vaccine is given to boys and girls around ages 11 or 12. The doses are given as a two-or three-part series over a six-month period depending on the age of the child.[15] The vaccine should be given before the child is sexually experimenting to benefit from its intended purpose of preventing HPV infection.

---

13 http://www.nccc-online.org/hpvcervical-cancer/cervical-cancer-overview (2016) Cervical cancer overview
14 https://www.cdc.gov/hpv/parents/cancer.html (2015) The link between HPV and cancer
15 http://www.cdc.gov/media/releases/2016/p1020-hpv-shots.html (2016) CDC recommends only two HPV shots for younger adolescents.

There are three vaccines currently available: Cervarix, Gardasil, and Gardasil-9. The difference between the three lies in the number of strains they fight. Gardasil-9 is the newest of the trio; it is effective against 9 strains of HPV rather than 2 or 4.[16]

According to the American Sexual Health Association, Gardasil "….is approximately 100% effective in preventing infection with HPV 6 and 11, which together are responsible for nearly all instances of genital warts." So yes, it works.[17]

As far as boosters go, once your child receives the series of two or three injections over six months, there is no need for a booster at this point. If your child only had one or two of the three doses, it is recommended that they receive the missed doses even if the six months have passed. They have until age 26 to do so.

The vaccine costs about $120 per dose for a total of $360. Most insurance companies cover the cost. However, if your insurance does not cover this, or if you do not have insurance, Gardasil participates in the Vaccine For Children (VFC) program. The VFC program will enable your child to receive the vaccine at no cost if your family meets certain requirements.[18]

Safety of Vaccines

Another mother wrote with concerns about safety. She stated:

"I never gave my girls the vaccine because I was very afraid of the long term effects. Because the vaccine was new, I didn't feel comfortable giving it them. Years later, I have heard some sad stories of side effects

---

16 http://www.cdc.gov/std/tg2015/hpv.htm (2016) Human Papillomavirus (HPV) infection

17 http://www.ashasexualhealth.org/stdsstis/hpv/hpv-vaccines (2016) HPV vaccines

18 https://www.gardasi_9.com/insurance-and-support/assistance-programs (2016) Assistance programs for those who aren't covered

that some girls developed because of the Gardasil vaccine (deregulates the immune system and causes viruses). It's scary to give your children vaccines and not knowing if you are helping them or making it worse."

Concerns over vaccine safety is common and understandable–after all, we are talking about the health of our children. I respect parents who take the time to find out all they can about vaccines.

According to a study released by the CDC's Morbidity and Mortality Weekly Report (Markowitz LE, Dunne EF, Saraiya M, et al. Human Papillomavirus Vaccination: Recommendations of the Advisory Committee on Immunization Practices (ACIP). MMWR Morb Mortal Wkly Rep. 2014;65(RR05):1-30.), the most common side effect is tenderness, swelling, and bruising at the injection site, dizziness after the injection is given, and skin infection at the injection site. I remember my daughters experiencing tenderness at the injection site which lasted a couple of days. If you have a big event in which your child is, say, pitching in a big game, you may want to reschedule around that. Otherwise, the side effects for the general population are no different than any other immunizations typically given to children.

If your child has had a previous allergic reaction to Gardasil or any other immunization, has an autoimmune disease, has a latex or yeast sensitivity, or is pregnant, it's best to talk to your healthcare provider to assess the risk/benefit to your child. It is likely the vaccine will not be given, depending on the circumstance. Keep in mind that anyone at any time can have a reaction to any immunization, but it is quite rare. Sort of like peanut butter or shellfish allergies; you do not withhold peanut butter from your child because you heard your neighbor's child reacted to peanut butter. Everyone is different.

Physicians are to report any adverse reactions of immunizations to the Vaccine Adverse Event Reporting System (VAERS), so anything unusual is documented and reported. For more information about the safety of the HPV vaccine, click on this link to the CDC to read about safety facts.

There are many scientific, well-researched reports on the safety of the HPV vaccine that conclude there are no severe side effects, even long-term.

What is the global perspective regarding HPV Vaccination?

I asked my daughter, who has a graduate degree in infectious disease, to offer her thoughts. She suggested I look at Australia's HPV prevention program–they are hugely successful in immunizing their population against HPV, unlike the United States. In the United States, only 37.6% of girls and 13.9% of boys completed their series of three immunizations in 2013.[19] In contrast, in the Land Down Under, 73.1% of girls and 60% of boys have completed their series, according to 2014 data.[20],[21] The difference? The Australian government felt the repercussions of HPV infection warranted a national program to offer free vaccines to all their 12–13-year-old students ... in school...at no cost. I'm not kidding. All students. Voluntary program. In school. Free. And parents said, "Heck, yes!" (Well, I'm not really sure anyone said that.)

There is currently a worldwide effort to vaccinate as many women as possible against HPV. The World Health Organization (WHO) supports global immunization. An organization called the Global Alliance for Vaccines and Immunizations or GAVI is currently

19 http://www.ashasexualhealth.org/hpv-vaccine-rates-are-up-but (2016) HPV vaccines rates are up, but...
20 http://www.hpvreg.ster.org.au/research/coverage-data/HPV-Vaccination-Coverage-2014 (2015) HPV vaccination coverage 2014
21 http://www.hpvregister.org.au/research/coverage-data/HPV-Vaccination-Coverage-2014–-Male (2015) HPV vaccination coverage 2014

introducing HPV vaccination programs worldwide.[22] However, other countries such as Hong Kong have a very low compliance rate.

Bottom line:

- HPV is a virus that is primarily transmitted through sexual contact.
- HPV is spread by skin-to-skin contact; therefore, a condom will not prevent the disease from spreading, but it may decrease the odds.
- Most adults will have HPV at some point in their lives.
- Most healthy immune systems naturally fight the virus off within two years.
- There are over 150 strains of HPV.
- Certain strains have been found to be the primary causes of genital warts and certain cancers. The cancers include cervical, penile, anal, vaginal, throat, and oral cancer.
- Oropharyngeal (throat, mouth) cancers rose 225% between 1998 and 2004 due to HPV according to the American Sexual Health Association[23].
- Vaccines are available for children starting at age 11 or 12.
- 99% of cervical cancer is caused by HPV.
- Since 2007, when the vaccine was first given, the HPV infection rate has decreased 56%.[24]
- 170,000,000 doses have been given worldwide according to the World Health Organization.[25]
- Always discuss any concerns about HPV and other vaccines with your healthcare provider.

---

22 http://www.gavi.org/support/nvs/human-papillomavirus (2016) Human papillomavirus vaccine support
23 http://ashasexualhealth.org/pdfs/HPV_Toolkit_2015.pdf (2015) The HPV Toolkit
24 http://www.ashasexualhealth.org/stdsstis/hpv/hpv-vaccines (2016) HPV vaccines
25 http://www.who.int/vaccine_safety/committee/topics/hpv/130619HPV_VaccineGACVSstatement.pdf (2013) GACVS Safety update on HPV Vaccines

Parents have the option to allow their child to be vaccinated against HPV. The best way to make an informed decision is to base your conclusions on research and evaluation and a consult with your healthcare provider. Use the links provided in this blog to read further. Next time you are discussing the pros and cons of vaccinating children against HPV at a party, take a sip of wine, smile and nod, and share your knowledge. Or change the topic to politics; certainly there are no conflicts on *that* topic, right?

World AIDS Day

When I was in nursing school in the very early 80s, we didn't learn about HIV/AIDS. We didn't know about it yet. I remember when the medical community began to discuss this new frightening disease, people were so quick to judge those who were diagnosed with it. And the fear of a child "catching" AIDS by attending the same school as another child who contracted it from a tainted blood transfusion...well, let's just say it was a scary movement. Granted, there was a lot of ignorance on everyone's part—we knew so little about it—but the public panic was pretty intense. I'm so glad we have a much better understanding of this disease now.

HIV stands for human immunodeficiency virus. (Now you know why we say HIV.) Typically, this virus is spread through bodily fluids, especially semen, blood, vaginal fluids, and rectal fluids. It is also spread by intravenous drug use (blood contact). Additionally, a mom can infect her baby during birth or by breastfeeding, though it is not as common.

Once a person has it, they can't get rid of it. Ever. There is no cure (right now). Some viruses, like the cold or flu, we eventually recover from and then are immune from it (well, that particular strain of it) for life. But with HIV, we are unable to fight it off.

When this virus enters a person's body, it starts to attack the cells that help us fight off infection (T cells). After a while, so many of these protective cells have been attacked that they can no longer effectively fight off infections. This is when HIV becomes AIDS—acquired immunodeficiency syndrome. At this point, a person is susceptible to "opportunistic" infections (OI)—infections that take advantage of this situation and attack the body. There are some pretty specific OI's associated with HIV, which healthcare providers use to diagnose AIDS. Unfortunately, this disease is terminal.

When a person is initially infected, they probably won't know it. If the person does have early symptoms (2-4 weeks after exposure), it feels like they are having a really nasty bout of the flu, but then after a couple weeks the person feels better. In fact, it could take up to ten years before the person feels sick again. And that is ten years that this person has been spreading HIV. Yikes. As has been mentioned before, get tested.

So, who are the people becoming infected? Here are some stats from the CDC from 2015:[26]

- 37% of new HIV infections are found in youth 20-29 years old.
- Over half of those are found in Hispanic/Latino and African-American gay or bisexual males.
- Men who have sex with men (MSM) account for 67% of all new HIV diagnoses.
- 24% of new diagnoses were attributed to heterosexual sex.
- 6% from IV drug use, and
- Most females (86%) contracted HIV through heterosexual sex, 13% from IV drug use. Overall, women accounted for 19% of HIV diagnoses in 2015.

In other words, anyone can get it even though certain demographics are at much higher risk.

On the positive side, there are medications that can put HIV-infected individuals into remission for a significant amount of time. This is

---

26 https://www.cdc.gov/hiv/statistics/overview/ataglance.html (2016) HIV in the United States: At A Glance

called antiretroviral treatment (ART) and must be used consistently.[27] Also, research is being done to come up with a vaccine against this fatal disease.

I want you to have a basic understand of HIV/AIDS so that you can understand why World AIDS Day, which is honored every December 1st, is so important.

"Shared Responsibility", part of the World Aids Day slogan, tells me that it is up to the educated sexual health community to ensure that people understand what this disease is and that no one is immune. It can happen to anybody. I do not know of one family who hasn't been touched by some type of terminal disease–cancer, Parkinson's, MS, Alzheimer's, and of course HIV/AIDS. Everyone deserves to be treated with dignity and respect no matter what their illness is. They deserve the best healthcare we can provide using the knowledge and medication available to us.

On World Aids Day, be that voice to support those who are facing a life with HIV/AIDS. Donate to your local AIDS organization, support research, be a positive voice for those battling this disease, learn more about HIV, get tested and/or encourage your loved ones to get tested as well. You can even participate in your local 5K to support AIDS research and support for those affected.

Initiate conversation with the young person in your life. Talk to them about what this disease is, and how to prevent it. (Abstain, use condoms–both male and female, get tested, don't share needles, shavers, or toothbrushes).

For more information go to AIDS.gov.

---

27 https://www.aids.gov/hiv-aids-basics/just-diagnosed-with-hiv-aids/treatment-options/overview-of-hiv-treatments/ (2015) Overview of HIV Treatments

The Best Defense Against HIV for Women and Girls: Education

Talking to our children about keeping healthy is one of the job requirements of parenting. From the minute they are fresh out of the oven, I mean womb, we immediately attach them to our breast. Heaven forbid they go too long without a nutritious meal.

From there it escalates. Frequent feedings, plenty of rest, bundling up our bundles of joy for security and warmth. As our children grow, we offer them healthy options at mealtime, ensure they have the appropriate clothing for the weather, and insist they wear bike helmets as they zoom into the world. Suddenly they are in middle school and making independent decisions about their health. You ponder, "Did I tell them everything they need to know so they will make wise decisions?" Well, probably not.

What was forgotten?

One topic that is oftentimes tossed aside until "later" is the conversation about human immunodeficiency virus, or HIV. Certainly that is a topic that is irrelevant during the middle school years, right?

Wrong.

Educating young people about HIV and other sexually transmitted infections (STIs) in middle school, before they become sexually active, is the best time to provide them with information and arm them with strategies to stay healthy before they are faced with sexual situations.

The CDC statistics about HIV speak for themselves.[28]

- Half of young people infected with HIV do not know they have it.[29]
- One-quarter of new HIV infections are diagnosed in the 13-24 year old age group, even though they reflect only 17% of the population.[30]
- The age group with the most HIV diagnoses (in 2013) were those aged 20-24.
- HIV is an "everyone" disease. Granted, most of those infected tend to be gay males, however females are not immune. In the United States, 1/4 of those with HIV are female, with 81% having contracted the disease within a heterosexual relationship.[31]

National Women and Girls HIV/AIDS Awareness Day is observed in March. Take time to focus on the following talking points with your daughters. However, the same conversations must be had with your sons. *Womenshealth.gov* is a terrific resource for more information.

- HIV is not AIDS (acquired immunodeficiency syndrome). HIV is the virus that causes AIDS. HIV can be treated, though not cured.
- Condoms can prevent the spread of HIV and some other STIs when used properly. Use condoms for anal, vaginal, and oral sex.
- HIV may not show any symptoms. Testing of both partners for HIV/STIs before beginning a sexual relationship is a must.
- Women contract HIV more easily than men. If a woman already has an STI, it also makes it easier to contract HIV.

---

28 http://www.cdc.gov/hiv/group/gender/women/index.html (2016) HIV Among Women
29 http://www.cdc.gov/hiv/group/age/youth/index.html (2016) HIV Among Youth
30 http://www.cdc.gov/hiv/group/age/youth/index.html (2016) HIV Among Youth
31 http://www.cdc.gov/hiv/group/age/youth/index.html (2016) HIV Among Youth

- HIV enjoys diverse populations; it does not discriminate on age, sex orientation, race, or ethnicity.
- For those at high-risk of contracting HIV from an infected partner, there are medications available. PrEP can help prevent HIV from infecting a person.[32] PEP is used to help lower your chances of getting HIV after exposure from an infected partner.[33]

Abstinence is the only 100% method to prevent HIV/STIs and pregnancy. However, using the following guidelines can help those who are sexually active stay healthy.

HIV/STI Prevention Basics: M.A.T.C.H.

1. When not abstinent, engage in a mutually **monogamous** relationship.
2. **Avoid** Alcohol and other drugs: People sometimes makes decisions they normally would not when sober. For proof, just listen to the Joe Nichols song, "Tequila Makes Her Clothes Fall Off."
3. Both partners should get **tested** for HIV and all STIs before sexual contact. Go to this CDC link to locate nearby testing facilities: https://gettested.cdc.gov.
4. Use a male or female **condom**…every time you have sex. Any kind of sex.

These four simple guidelines can help those who are sexually active stay **healthy**.

Finally, be nice to those who have HIV. There is no place for bullying and teasing in this world.

---

32 https://www.aids.gov/hiv-aids-basics/prevention/reduce-your-risk/pre-exposure-prophylaxis/ (2016) Pre-exposure Prophylaxis (PrEP)
33 http://www.cdc.gov/hiv/basics/pep.html (2016) Post-exposure Prophylaxis (PEP)

For more information about HIV/AIDS, the following resources are excellent.

Womenshealth.gov
CDC.gov
aids.govWorld Health Organization
Avert.org

What Will You Tell Your Child Today? Twelve Talking Tips about HIV/AIDS

Because it is expected that you communicate with your kids or other youth in your lives about sexuality health, having medically-accurate information about HIV/AIDS is crucial in understanding the landscape of this disease.

HIV, or human immunodeficiency virus, is spread via bodily fluids such as semen, vaginal fluids, blood, and breast milk. Take note that saliva is *not* on that list. These fluids are then transferred to the next person by coming into contact with another person's blood or mucus membranes (mouth, vagina, rectum, or tip of the penis.) Having unprotected sex is the primary method of infection, so using a condom correctly is clearly one way to be protected. A person cannot contract HIV from toilet seats, shaking hands, sharing beverages, hugging, or drinking from water fountains.

HIV is a virus that the body cannot get rid of, unlike other viruses such as the cold or flu bug. This virus likes to stick around and attack the immune system. As HIV continues to attack, it also replicates itself, which allows the virus to attack the immune system further. After a while, usually about ten years without treatment, the body is no longer able to fight even simple infections and the diagnosis of AIDS is made.

AIDS, or acquired immunodeficiency syndrome, is considered the final stage of HIV and is typically fatal after about three years.[34] For more information about HIV/AIDS, go to AIDS.gov.[35]

---

34 https://www.aids.gov/hiv-aids-basics/hiv-aids-101/what-is-hiv-aids/ (2016) What is HIV/AIDS?

35 https://www.aids.gov/hiv-aids-basics/hiv-aids-101/what-is-hiv-aids/ (2016) What is HIV/AIDS?

The good news is, there is testing available to determine if you or your partner have HIV/AIDS. Antiretroviral therapy (ART) is a combination of medications that can help prevent HIV from progressing to AIDS and allow a person to live a full life.[36]

Even though today is an awareness day for women and girls, males should not be excluded from the conversation; 86% of women are infected by their male partners.[37]

HIV/AIDS is an "every person" discussion. Whether your child identifies as gay or straight, bisexual or transgender, it is imperative they have information that can protect them. Knowing and understanding about the disease and prevention BEFORE they are sexually active is the best way to arm them with the tools they need to have safer sex.

Nationally, only 33% of our schools require HIV/AIDS education.[38] It is important for you to have the discussion about this and other STIs with your children.

Starting the conversation

Take advantage of conversation opportunities such as riding in the car (captive audience!), taking them on a walk or out to dinner, or in the stillness of the night before they go to sleep. Rather than just blurting out "I don't want you to get AIDS!" try a more gentle approach. "Can we talk?" Pretty simple. Now that you have their attention, explain that you just happened to be reading about HIV/AIDS and would like to share what you learned. Ask them if they

---

36 https://www.aids.gov/hiv-aids-basics/just-diagnosed-with-hiv-aids/treatment-options/overview-of-hiv-treatments/ (2015) Overview of HIV Treatments

37 http://www.cdc.gov/hiv/statistics/overview/ataglance.html (2016) HIV in the United States: *At A Glance*

38 http://www.ncsl.org/research/health/state-policies-on-sex-education-in-schools.aspx (2015) State Policies on Sex Education in Schools

have talked about it in school and if they can share insights with you as well. This ensures they are involved in this conversation and it does not become a lecture.

The following are facts that can inspire conversation. One conversation about HIV/AIDS–or any other important life topic–should be discussed often and over the course of time. Therefore, no need to hit on all the following facts at once, but they will give you a few talking points.

The following information is found on Womenshealth.gov.[39]

1. Of all the people who live with HIV, 25% are women.
2. 80% of those women are age 15-44.
3. 25% do not seek medical care because of many barriers.
4. Only half are receiving medical care for HIV, and only 40% of those women have it under control.
5. Abstinence is the only way to fully prevent HIV. However, using a condom correctly with vaginal, anal, and oral sex can help reduce the risk.
6. Your partner and yourself should get tested before engaging in sexual activity and as part of your annual checkup. Most STI's and HIV do not show obvious symptoms right away.
7. Get yourself tested (GYT) for STI's as well. Having an STI increases your risk of contracting HIV.
8. Casual contact or toilet seats will not expose you to AIDS.
9. Alcohol and drugs increases risky behavior. Which increases your odds for not using a condom. Which increases your odds of contracting an STI or AIDS.
10. Do not share needles or syringes with another person.
11. Your risk of HIV is influenced by many factors, including your partners' history. Don't be afraid to have the conversation about past drug use or sexual history. Even so, get tested together.

39 https://www.womenshealth.gov/hiv-and-aids (2016) HIV and AIDS

12. As always, if you ever have questions about HIV, STI's or other sexual health issues, never hesitate to approach your healthcare provider.

Finally, be a kind, compassionate global citizen and show support for those who live with HIV/AIDS. Donate to your local AIDS Foundation, participate in fundraisers or walks, educate peers about HIV facts, and show support for those you may meet someday with HIV/AIDS.

"Daddy, put your big penis on." Preschool son to his dad after a particularly cold shower.

"Mommy doesn't normally wear handcuffs or a blindfold." A dad describing an unfortunate 'unlocked door' situation.

"I have been there through those "character building" moments with my children. If you are there for your child, listen and encourage, you often find they come out of the situation stronger!!" Mom of two.

PARENT SUPPORT:

parenthood isn't sainthood

We All Need a Little Help

On Friday night I enjoyed a glass (or two) of relaxing red wine and scrumptious cheese in our lovely city. The best part of the evening was the candid conversation I had with a close friend of mine, Mary.

Mary told me that a friend of hers had dealt with exactly what this book is dedicated to–adolescent sexuality health. Her friend's daughter was in high school at the time, and even though there was no reason to believe her daughter was sexually active at that time, she wanted to be sure her daughter took the appropriate precautions in the event that were to change.

This woman had a close relationship with her daughter, but understanding that kids are not always comfortable talking with their parents about sex, she explained to Mary that she had appointed her as her daughter's "go to" person if she ever had any questions, problems, or needs regarding her sexual health. No questions asked.

Mary conveyed she felt deeply honored to be entrusted to another woman's child for such an important role.

I thought to myself that this is one of the most loving things a parent can do. As parents, we want to know EVERYTHING that is going on with our child. After all, WE were the ones who gave birth or went through the adoption process! A lot of love, pain, tears, MONEY went into getting our kids into this world…and we want to be a part of every step. But to be willing to take a step back and tell your daughter or son that you only want them healthy and safe–and that you are willing to allow another trusted adult to be that person for them if needed–is such a wonderful gift. I'm guessing that that gesture alone probably secured a trust between that parent and child.

So, if you find yourself in a position in which you feel you need a little help from your friends, don't be afraid to ask. That is an incredibly responsible thing to do for your child.

Dedicated Dads

A dad is *that guy* who is traditionally seen as someone who works diligently all day to earn a living for his beloved family. However, we all know that what is known as "the traditional family" is morphing into a variety of perfectly acceptable variations: single-parent, two moms, two dads, step-parents, grandparents, guardians…you name it. It's all good! However, for the purpose of this writing, I am going to use the word "dad" meaning any man that is a consistent and visible presence in a child's world. It could be a birth dad, step dad, grand dad, uncle, family friend…you know who you are.

So men, you think the women in your lives want you to communicate more??? Now researchers want you to be more communicative, too–with your kids. Yes, it is time to man-up and communicate with your children.

It matters. Just ask Tim. He is quite certain he ruined his son; you may agree after you read this:

How I ruined my son…

> *"My son used to hang out with me when I was in the shower.*
> *I did not realize how observant he was…*
> *One day (maybe after a colder shower… LOL) he said, 'Daddy put your big penis on.'*
> *Looking back, I should have had a discussion with him. He was about 3 or 4 yrs old."*

Or maybe his son ruined him? I'm not sure. But what a great teachable moment! In the shower, talking about penis size. Hey–you take those moments when you get them!

Or possibly your child will teach you something, as the same dad reminisced about this moment with his daughter:

How I ruined my daughter...

"I was in the basement sorting laundry. My younger daughter was helping me... she was probably about 12 or so...
I came across what I thought was "thong underwear."
I asked with alarm and concern "Whose the heck are these?" She said that they were hers.
I was shocked. I was expecting to be told that they belonged to her older sister.
When she said that they belonged to her, I got really concerned and actually frightened.. it probably showed in the tone and level of my voice...
My next question was "Where did you get these?" which she answered "Mom."
"Mom?" I responded... She followed with "What's the big deal Dad?" Her embarrassment was increasing as my anger was increasing.
I then said "Do you know what this is?" and she with a high level of embarrassment said "yes, a training bra."
Ouch...
To her credit, she continued to help me sort laundry after that..."

Even though this dad received a brutal lesson in becoming competent in adolescent undergarments (maybe a field trip to Victoria's Secret should be on his agenda next??), the lessons his daughter received were even more valuable:

- He broke gender stereotypes by doing "women's work" (???)
- His daughter learned the value (and human connection) of working with others.
- She learned that her dad did NOT want her wearing dental-floss, I mean, thong underwear at a young age.

- Finally, she learned that maybe next time she will volunteer to clean toilets instead...

Many family values were shared in that moment. Awesome, if you ask me.

Ah, yes. Communication...

Vincent Guilamo-Ramos, a professor at NYU Silver School of Social Work, along with some peers from the CDC, analyzed several studies regarding the relationship between a "paternal" figure (dad, stepdad, granddad, uncle, etc.) and the adolescent in their life and how it impacted the young person's sexual decision-making. In this enlightening report, published in *Pediatrics*, they found a few consistent implications as they analyzed these studies.[1]

The bottom line is, dads (or father figures) who connect with, who communicate with, and who have a genuine attachment to their kids can positively influence the young person in their life when it comes to sexual decision-making. Having conversations about expectations when it comes to sex isn't always easy. Yet, it has been found that the child will be more likely to delay the first time they have sex, will be more likely to use a condom, and less likely to engage in risky sexual behavior.

Here's a great example from Dave P. who wrote:

> *"I have a stepdaughter, age 16, who has started dabbling in "experimentation" with members of the opposite sex, mainly what my generation would call "playing kissy face" with boys. One such incident occurred last summer when, after GPS-*

---

1   Paternal Influences on Adolescent Sexual Risk Behaviors: A Structured Literature Review Vincent Guilamo-Ramos, Alida Bouris, Jane Lee, Katharine McCarthy, Shannon L. Michael, Seraphine Pitt-Barnes, Patricia Dittus Pediatrics Nov 2012, 130 (5) e1313-e1325; **DOI:** 10.1542/peds.2011-2066

ing her phone, I discovered her in a parked car in a not-so-nearby park with a boy that was about 3 years older. This jarred my memory about my own "good times" when I was a teen. But then I realized that life and sexual encounters today aren't quite like they used to be. Kids are having sex at much younger ages these days and may not be as aware of the need for protection. The general mentality of today's teens seems to demonstrate a feeling of "immortality" and that nothing is going to happen to them.

When my wife and I sat down with "Angie," and discussed boys, their not-so-hidden agendas, and the need for protection, she was quite put off, stating she was well aware of all this. I advised her she shouldn't use sex to get someone's attention (which this clearly was), and that it should be something that's shared between two people that have strong feelings for each other. They don't think about reputation or the harm it could potentially do to their bodies. As I explained, we are looking out for her own well-being. She understood and seems to have taken this advice to heart (or so I think!). As a step-father, discussing things like this with her, as well as my stepson (15 yrs), has allowed me to feel closer to them and create a stronger overall bond within the family."

See! Open communication works! Not only did these parents use this opportunity to teach about healthy vs. unhealthy relationships, they used the opportunity to share their values. Having a value system in place helps build self-efficacy which in turn inspires young people to delay having sex for the first time.

Then again, maybe there are times when putting up a barrier (ie: locked door) would be more useful, as Bob H. recollects:

"My son walked in on my wife and I in the midst of wild romance…he closed the door and exclaimed, "I don't believe

I just saw what I just saw..."
We explained that Mommy doesn't normally wear handcuffs
or a blindfold...
Honestly...I just sat him down and explained when a door
is closed he needs to always knock. What Mom and I were
doing was sharing something that a man and a woman both
need and enjoy. He was ok with everything. He did say he
preferred if we would lock the door because he wasn't going
to remember to knock, and he still couldn't believe we still did
that stuff...that was 10-12 years ago...LOL Hysterical...we
all three still laugh."

Having a sense of humor about sexuality is a great ice-breaker. It can reassure the child that it is okay to talk about this stuff with dad (or mom) and that adults actually "get it." They will see you as a safe person to talk with–and isn't that what you want?

Using time with your child to communicate personal values has proven beneficial. However, educating one's son or daughter can also be beneficial when having one of these heart-to-heart conversations about sex.

Here's what one dad had to say:

"When my son reached middle school age, my wife decided
that it was time for me to have a discussion with him about sex.
While we had private discussions, one memorable exchange
came during a talk that included my son's close friend and his
father. My wife thought it might be helpful to have a 'two Dad
–two son' discussion, and that it might be more comfortable
for all. Rather than lecturing, I decided it might be interesting
to try to discover what the boys already knew. So I asked open
ended questions. What did they know about reproduction?
What did they know about conception? And so on... We were

*caught off guard a bit because we got pretty candid answers.
And it was clear that they already had some good information
about puberty, reproduction, and even some aspects of birth
control and sexually transmitted diseases. However, nothing
could have prepared us for the response when the discussion
turned to more specifics about sexual contact.*
Q: What do you know about oral sex?
*A: (Without hesitation both boys said nearly in unison) Oh
that's when you do it over the phone!*
*My advice to parents–assume nothing. Ask. You will be
amazed by the answers you get."*

Ahhh…never assume your kids already know this stuff. Great
advice, Dad. And I especially love the technique to assess what the
kids already knew first. Kudos!

One final thought from Tim S., a father of four.

*"I never really talked with my dad much at all… I was blessed
to have a wife that was wise enough and comfortable enough
to talk with the kids about sex at a very early age explaining
to them "how things work." It was not a "Big Talk" but just
conversations that came up during the day, etc… I was part
of that conversation…I did attempt to make the distinction
of the difference between sexual feelings and love. As a
young person, I was pretty confused not understanding the
difference, or knowing there was a difference."*

The difference between love and sex. What a wonderful conversation
that would be with your child, especially as they are beginning to
experience all those confusing feelings that come with puberty and
hormonal influx. Thanks, Tim.

I think you get the idea. These dads set about to address only one topic, or merely wanted to fold laundry, yet ended up addressing a variety of pertinent sex topics. As you confidently (well, just fake it) embark on a series of sexual health conversations, you may find yourself discussing topics with your kids that you did not plan on, just as these dads experienced. Little did they realize what they were actually teaching their children....

- Anatomy (Penis shrinkage–hey! It's a fact of life!)
- Mechanics of sex (Well, we can call it physiology if that makes you nervous.)
- Appropriate expressions of love
- Sex is private (i.e.: Please don't sext!)
- Relationships: Love vs Sex
- Healthy vs. Unhealthy relationships
- Sexual terminology
- Undergarments. Well, okay–maybe that is something that isn't necessarily pressing.

One other interesting finding from the study: It seems that young people with super strict parents or super lenient parents tend to engage in sex earlier than those with parents who were more middle-of-the-road. I bet that little tidbit has your wheels spinning now, doesn't it?

As you make time for the young person in your life, turn off your phone and put it away. Give them 100% attention. This not only tells the child that you care deeply for them, but that what you are about to discuss is very important. They will not only listen, but they will *hear* you. And we all want our kids to hear our voices in their head as they enter the throes of ecstasy with their (current) love-of-their-life, right? That oughta kill the mood.

To read more, these articles are informative:

http://www.clafh.org/news-and-events/18/ (2012) Center for Latino Adolescent and Family Health Study Finds That Fathers Matter When It Comes to Their Teenager's Sexual Behavior

https://www.ncbi.nlm.nih.gov/pubmed/24549437 (2014) A Qualitative Analysis of Father–Son Relationships among HIV-Positive Young Black Men Who Have Sex with Men

---

Car Accidents and Healthy Relationships: Ten Realizations that Evolve from Being Un–Dead

Relationships are the backbone of our mental, emotional and social well-being. Many times we take our friends and family for granted. We may not always appreciate how loved we are—or how much we love and care for others, until something happens. Let me share with you a personal experience that prompted a little introspection on my part.

Being the longest. winter. ever. in Illinois a couple of years ago, we unexpectedly endured a late season snowfall. The city forgot to use protection to prevent accidents; no plows or salt trucks to be seen… nor was the ice beneath the snow visible. Those of us who prefer to not grapple with our car being forced into an unforgiving ditch, we patiently drove white-knuckled along the road, inch by inch.

I was poking along at half the posted speed, steering wheel clutched, when I noticed a car in the oncoming lane begin to fishtail. I watched in disbelief as the car advanced closer, closer, closer gaining momentum with each swerve—my car as the target.

"This is not going to end well," I thought solemnly.

Grasping the steering wheel tighter, I took a deep breath and braced as the missile-on-wheels crossed the center lane–directly into my path. I do not remember the moment of impact, which is probably a good thing, however I do remember hesitantly opening my astonished eyes with the realization:

I. Am. Not. Dead.

Smelling something oddly suspicious of smoke (which turned out to be eau-de-airbag), I grabbed my purse (my phone!) and ran out into the snow. Soon paramedics, police, and firetrucks arrived (how *did* they get there so fast?) and I was whisked off to the ER with only minor airbag injuries. Thankfully, the other stunned driver was okay as well. However, both our heroic cars lost their dependable lives saving ours.

Alas, one more example to reiterate this fact: *use protection.*

As soon as I was able, I sent a text to two friends–whom I knew to be driving on the perilous roads–to alert them to the road conditions via a photo of my totaled car: "Roads are bad."

Within minutes my phone was lighting up with texts. "Are you okay?" "What happened?" "How can I help?"

Relationships: Ten Realizations that Evolve When One is Delightfully Un-dead
OR…
What I Learned from Being in a Super Scary Car Crash

1. **First, thank the car.** The relationship you have with your airbag and seatbelt is one of sacrifice and support–yet they expect nothing in return. *Use them*–you never know when you will need them. It is the one relationship in which it is okay to take advantage of their unrequited goodness.
2. **Kindness and compassion enhance pain relief.** The evening of my accident, a cherished friend stopped by to present me with three essential items guaranteed to bring immediate healing: a ginormous bouquet of flowers, a ginormous box of Godiva, and a ginormous bottle of grapefruit vodka. All three ginormous treats helped bring emotional healing, but none more than her ginormous, spirited presence.

3. **There's nothing like a hug.** There are many mechanisms to maintain relationships: Facebook, Face Time, texting, emails, phone, letters, and old-fashioned coffee dates all have a part in our crazy, tech-driven world. In an instant, you can be connected with loved ones around the world and can even see their smiling faces while exploring far-away continents. But there is nothing like the hug of a friend to feel connected.

   As a young nursing student, I was taught about a phenomenon, failure-to-thrive, in which infants actually died because they were not being held. Adults also need that human touch to thrive in our world. Free hugs anyone?

4. **Friends want to be there.** Some people will drop everything to pick up a bewildered friend and give them a lift home. Of course, this involved a comedy-of-errors-afternoon trying to locate my totaled car in an unknown location to retrieve my personal belongings. It was actually a sad moment.

5. **Relationships are as unique as the individuals who form them.** The people we choose, yes choose, to be in our lives offer us something uniquely special to enhance our life journey. Hopefully we do the same for them. Balance is key. We may have a dear friend who holds an opposing view on certain issues, yet their goodness and kindness shines through to allow for an unexpected kinship. The mutual respect allows for laughter and an agreement to disagree. Life is too short to not appreciate differences and embrace friendships with people who offer something new to our world.

6. **Physical pain stinks, but so does emotional pain.** Physical discomfort takes some time to heal. However, as the adrenalin dissipated, and the realization of the severity of the accident hit, tears suddenly flowed days later. I had a friend who hopped at the opportunity to hold me when the frightened tears finally released.

7. **Our children really *do* like us!** You know those rolling eyeballs I refer to on occasion? One day the eyeballs will refocus to what is really important (you, of course). But it is up to you, their first and most important teacher, to show them how to love unconditionally.

8. **One of the most important relationships you have is with yourself**, because in the end, that is who you are stuck with. Care for yourself, do what makes your soul happy. You will find people who cross your path who are meant to be in your world at the right time in the right place.
9. **You will always be your parent's baby.** Don't believe me? Make the phone call that starts with, "I'm okay, but I need you to know..."
10. **Grab an amazing friend and get out of Dodge.** Escape once in a while. Whether it be to the movies, dinner, or a trip across the country looking for the elusive summer, change your perspective. Get your tarot cards read (hey, you *know* your future is bright! You are a survivor!), walk in the sand, enjoy a decadent dessert... because life is good. Enjoy each day. Do not take your moments for granted.

Healthy relationships are the crux of good health. A supportive, caring community of humans—whether it be one or two close friends or a large circle of individuals—build you up as a person, strengthen you when down, and help you to see the world through interesting and varied eyes. When we care for ourselves we are able to accept care from others, and are then able to build trust to allow us to love fully and completely.

We will all have to face moments of darkness such as accidents, cancer, or divorce. The people in our lives will allow us to move forward with their support. These are the same people who will celebrate with you the amazing joys that life brings as well. Embrace these relationships.

Legacy: What Ann Taught Me

Legacy.

When we consider legacy, our thoughts often meander to "The Greats:" The legacy of spectacular athletes, the legacy of effective presidents, the legacy of prestigious universities.

Yet, the most empowering legacies are left by those who are in our daily lives; our parents, children, co-workers, teachers, and friends.

Today I am honoring a close friend who journeyed through the valleys and mountains of the Big C. As I reflect on the past several years of Ann's skirmishes and all-out armed warfare against this unforgiving enemy, my discombobulated thoughts return to one thing: her legacy.

Walking into her room at hospice this week, I was overwhelmed with the sense of love and bonding between the five remarkable daughters sitting by her side. The alliance they formed while their worlds transitioned appeared to be an unspoken vow to their mom...

"We got this, Mom. You taught us. It's okay."

Legacy? You bet. Despite all the typical "sister issues" every family experiences, it is clear Ann left a legacy of love and unwavering commitment to the care and well-being of each other, each sister. It was palpable. It was powerful.

This immense sense of goodness offered an opportunity for me to reflect on the legacy Ann left for me personally. It also gave pause to consider what I hope to leave for my own children.

Before her initial diagnosis, Ann and I enthusiastically volunteered to hand out water at the 13.1 mile water station of the Chicago Marathon. As we awkwardly shoved water cups into the hands of dedicated runners, we entertained ourselves with ongoing comments that reflected the idea that—if *they* can do it, we can *totally* do it. Bad-ass runner-talk commenced and plans were instantly made.

Then came her diagnosis of breast cancer…dashing our bad-ass plans.

However, I went on to run 26.2 the next year. In fact, she ran with me—her name on an American Cancer Society ribbon flapping in the wind off my backside.

Over ten years have gone by since then. Many races have been run, many donations have been made, many tears have been shed. But I promise, no one I have met has run a race quite like Ann.

What were the legacies she left with me and other friends?

- Strength, endurance, and hope. She was a petite, wisp of a woman who fought with superhuman strength. If she can do that, then I can do this.
- Life is short. Go out and have adventures…before you can't.
- Pick a few close friends and love them fiercely.
- Don't worry what other people think of you, just be your own awesome cool self. (And trust me, she was cool!)
- Take time to reflect on the legacy you hope to leave for your tribe of loved ones.

Consider conversations with our children and what an impact you can make, especially when addressing sexuality health issues.

- Are your conversations respectful? You will leave them with a legacy of respecting others for who they are.
- Are your conversations encouraging? You will leave a legacy of reaching for the stars and fulfilling hopes and dreams. Give it a shot! There is no true success without effort.
- Are your conversations honest? You will leave a legacy in which it is okay for your loved ones to express themselves confidently and the ability to actively listen to others when they are sharing.
- Are your conversations humorous? You will have a legacy of joy by taking life a little less seriously.
- Are your conversations open? You leave a legacy that opinions can be shared respectfully. It is okay to agree to disagree. But remember, you never know what you will learn from someone else's views.
- Finally, have conversations with your children ended a bit...angrily? That's okay—it happens to all of us. Follow up with an "I'm sorry." This will leave a legacy of humility.

I asked some parents what kind of legacy they hope to leave for their children. Here are their thoughtful responses:

Matt Mason:

"I would want to be someone they could look up to, that they could be proud of and say, "My dad was a hard worker and a good husband." I want to be a light to them when the world seems dark. I may not always live that way, but I try my best to be an example they can be proud of."

Dawn Joyce-Meier:

- *"Embrace life!*
- *Live each day to its fullest!*

- *Live, Love, Laugh*
- *Be Kind*
- *Make a difference!*
- *Make time for family and friends!*
- *Accept yourself and love who you are!*
- *Travel the world!"*

Sue Bowman:
"I hope my children know that there will never be another person in their life who thinks about them every day, prays for them and loves them unconditionally as I do. I read a quote the other day that I loved. 'There is never anyone so far beneath you that you can't learn something from and no one so far above you that you need permission to communicate with them.'"

Nancy Stanis:
" I had the following "rules to live by" on my refrigerator as my children were growing up. I think my kids have taken these rules to heart and live them every day in their adult lives."

It is not OK....
*to look down on people who are poor or powerless,
to laugh at people because of the way they look or dress,
to make fun of people who speak with accents,
to disparage people because of their sexual orientation,
to ignore people who have disabilities,
to stereotype people based on gender, race or nationality,
to deride people's religious, political or personal beliefs,
to mistake opinions for understanding,
...attitudes for wisdom,
...or self-righteousness for truth
to believe that we are more-or less-important than anyone.*
It is OK...
to be less than perfect,

to be fallible,
to be human,
as long as we try honestly each day to love our neighbors as
ourselves-for the love of God.

Pam Smith
"*A legacy of faith.*"

Kelly Kelley
"*Ralph Waldo Emerson expresses my thoughts. 'What lies*
behind us and what lies before us are small matter compared
to what lies within us. And when we bring what is within us
out into the world, miracles happen.'"

And for my daughters, what do I want *my* legacy to be?

- One of kindness and compassion towards all people: a kind word and friendly smile can make a difference in someone's day.
- An understanding that no one is perfect, including ourselves
- Wonderment of the world and the beautiful people who live in it
- To live their authentic lives (as long as they invite me along on the journey!)
- And to take care of their bodies to live a long and vigorous life

Finally…a legacy of love. Because, my friend, at the end of our journey, nothing else matters.

Legacy. Make it personal. What do you hope will be your legacy to the loved ones in your world?

National Women's Health Week: Dimensions of Wellness

May is a busy month! Not only do we have Mother's Day and *National Teen Pregnancy Prevention Week*, it is also *National Women's Health Week* as promoted by the *Office of Women's Health (Womenshealth. gov)*.

It is important for everyone to take care of themselves. However, it is my observation that many women put their health on the back burner. When our children are younger, it often feels as if our wheels are spinning: meals, activities, work, volunteering, housekeeping, maintaining relationships. It takes significant time out of our day. To schedule one. more. thing on our calendar seems daunting.

As we get older and our children are flying the coop, one would think free time would be available in spades. I am here to tell you that is not necessarily true. All of a sudden, we find ourselves filling our calendar with more of the same–sans children. How does that happen? I do not have the answer to that; I am often left wondering what happened to my days. The old adage "time moves faster as you get older" is absolutely true. Yet, our health should have a prominent place at the top of our priority list.

Why is it important we stay on top of our health?

Coming from a nursing background, I am a huge proponent of preventative medicine. If we vaccinate, we can prevent serious illness such as influenza and meningitis. If we visit the dermatologist, we can find those pesky little pre-cancerous spots before they become disfiguring or worse. If we visit the dentist, we can prevent gum disease which can affect the health of our entire body, not just our mouth. In other words, by occasionally taking a small amount of time out of your day to visit with various health care providers, you could ultimately be saving yourself time, money, and heartache down the road.

But, living a life of wellness is more than visiting the doctor annually or putting out that cigarette. Wellness is an integration, or blending, of many well-being dimensions. They work together to create a healthy balance of the many facets of our lives. The blending of these dimensions is what enables individuals to maintain good health. It is up to us, as individuals, to take charge of our wellness with the choices we make.

I thought I would take a moment to share what I do to maintain a level of wellness in each dimension. How many can you relate to?

Dimensions of Wellness

Physical Wellness

Keep regular medical appointments for your dermatologist, dentist, primary care physician, gynecologist, and any other doc you routinely visit. Get that colonoscopy and mammogram as directed by your healthcare provider. I schedule my gynecologist appointment the same month as my birthday each year—I am guaranteed to remember to make that appointment. Good heath is a gift to myself.

Exercise regularly. I make it a habit to workout with my friends; not only do they keep me accountable, but my workout becomes play time. It not only boosts a person physically but socially and emotionally as well.

Limit alcohol intake. Well, at least try. Okay, so today was a bad day. There's always tomorrow. Best to keep it at a drink a day, however.[2]

Do not smoke. If you do smoke, do not smoke around other people. Second-hand smoke stinks.[3] I am pretty adamant about this; my dad, a non-smoker, died very young of lung cancer. Please do not put me at risk, too.

Emotional Wellness

Having the ability to understand our own emotions and finding healthy outlets for those feelings helps us cope with daily issues. Finding friends to confide in, exercising, writing our feelings down, and talking to therapists are all healthy ways of recognizing and coping with our emotions.

I have found a lovely circle of friends with whom I can be myself with, but only a select few that I share my most intimate thoughts. Sharing sorrows and joys—frustrations and celebration with others helps us cope effectively. I also feel better after a relaxing walk or vigorous run. Screaming and yelling may feel good for that brief second but is highly ineffective. Not that I would know...

Intellectual Wellness

Keep your mind stimulated by learning something new every day, whether it is related to your professional interests or your personal interests. Be sure to fill your mind with stuff that is true and accurate...with the exception of fiction movies and books. Nothing like a little escapism to maintain your emotional wellness.

---

2   http://www.cdc.gov/alcohol/fact-sheets/alcohol-use.htm (2016) Alcohol Use and Your Health
3   http://www.cdc.gov/tobacco/data_statistics/fact_sheets/secondhand_smoke/general_facts/index.htm (2016) Secondhand Smoke (SHS) Facts

I spend my days writing, discussing, and reading information based on my occupation. I stay connected with others who share my intellectual interests. I also enjoy reading books of all varieties to keep my mind open to new ideas. I love a good story!

You don't want to nourish your mind with junk information any more than you want to nourish your body with junk food.

Social Wellness

Maintain a close circle of friends. Having people to connect with and share your world with is an amazing gift you give yourself. Support systems enable people to navigate through life's highs and lows.

I have a few different circles of friends that I enjoy spending time with. Book club, work friends, Bunko nights, running girls, workout girls…they all add something to my world. Reach out to others who you know may not have those connections. Start a book club or enjoy a coffee break once a month with someone new.

Spiritual Wellness

Spiritual moments may occur in many environments: church, on a walk in the woods, while meditating, on a run. Spirituality is a personal thing. It helps people stay grounded and enables them retain their focus on what is important in their lives.

I find my most spiritual moments are when I am running alone and have time to contemplate. I feel refreshed and energized.

Occupational Wellness

Whether your job is maintaining a household or running a corporation, never think for a moment what you do is not appreciated and needed.

If you feel fulfilled by your work and are able to reasonably balance your life, you are in a healthy place.

I spend my time researching and writing about topics I feel are important and timely. My passion is educating and sharing with others so they feel empowered with information. I want them to feel they are not alone in their parenting journey.

Environmental Wellness

Living and working in an environment in which a person feels safe and comfortable is conducive to well-being. Have you noticed recently that nurses, while taking your medical history, will quiz you about the safety within your home? They want to be sure you are living in a healthy environment.

As a citizen of my environment, I ensure my home is clean, safe, and pleasant for my family. Most of the time. Okay, sometimes.

Remember to practice habits that enable you to live a life of balanced wellness. You are modeling this behavior for your children. They may appear oblivious to your lifestyle, but wait until they are adults and see what happens. Little snippets of you start shining though. For better or worse. Or both.

Support Other Women: Talk Behind Their Backs

Recently I attended a women's entrepreneurial event in Chicago. I met some pretty awesome and inspiring women: driven, emerging adults as well as self-actualized, grown-ass women. Whether these incredible women are finding their way developing their businesses or making seven figures, the common theme that permeated the environment was …

LIFT UP and SUPPORT other women. No, this is not a bra ad. Do not view women as competition, but rather seek them out as a complement to your own world. We see it all the time. We judge others on appearance, income, career, lifestyle, friends, children, and even their personality. Often we judge others because we envy them, but that can instill an unhealthy and untrue view about the people we envy—and about ourselves! This is so important to acknowledge when we are addressing adolescent sexual health.

One crucial issue to discuss with our children is the concept of healthy relationships. Typically, we hone in on romantic relationships, but friendships and eventually professional relationships have a significant influence on our mental, emotional, and social health.

Social media has done a tremendous disservice to the population at large when it comes to encouraging envy. Explain to our daughters and sons that what one sees on social media is not a true reflection of what is real in each of our lives.

I have a friend who frequently comments that I never take a bad photo as evidenced by Facebook. Well, let me tell you, most of my photos are bad—but am I going to post those? Heck, no! Do I post photos of me in my grungy clothes, no make-up, reading glasses askew, messy hair, flab hanging out while I slump over a computer all day? Heck, no! That is my real-world reality. As I view photos my friends post about the fun they are having, the friends they are with, the trips they are enjoying, I understand they are no different than I am! They are merely posting exceptional moments in their lives, not the daily ho-hum world we all live in.

We need to be sure our children understand that no one person is any "better" or any "worse" comparatively. Just different. And these differences are what add dimension to our lives. Wasting time envying another person only serves to drag us down.

You are a role model. No matter your income level, whether or not you are employed, or even if you may or may not have children; there are young girls watching you, learning from you and forming ideas about the world based on their observations of you. Be a strong upstanding individual who talks about others, especially women, behind their backs. Yes, you heard me. This is the kind of stuff we need to be saying:

"She has a kind heart."
"She works so hard."
"She is a special friend."
"She looks amazing—her workouts have paid off!"
"She is someone I admire."
"She's come through some tough times—she is remarkable."

Am I so perfect? Ah, no. It is so easy to get caught up in negative conversation (i.e. gossip). But each time I bite my tongue, I sleep a little easier.

I challenge my readers to be an example for your daughters (and sons!) and support other women in your world. Talk about them behind their backs. Ask your daughters about the super cool qualities they see in their friends and family, especially if they start complaining about them! No one is perfect, but we can certainly focus on the good qualities we all have.

You, my dear readers, are pretty awesome! I really appreciate how much you care about the young people in your world and truly want to make a difference in their lives.

International Kissing Day

July 6 is International Kissing Day. No need to allow this so-very-important-day to pass by without celebration! Give your child a kiss on their rosy cheek, on top of their head, or tip of their nose. Below are a few additional suggestions to recognize Kissing Day.

1. Share a funny memory of one of your very first awkward kisses. This allows your child to realize 'awkward' is normal. More importantly, it serves as a conversation starter for more serious topics about relationships.
2. Compare and contrast different types of relationships: families, friends, acquaintances, romantic partners, and relationships in which an adult holds a position of power, such as a coach or teacher.
3. Ask your child which type of kiss or other expressions of affection are appropriate for which type of relationship? A peck on the cheek? A kiss on the hand? A hug? A smile?
4. Discuss consent. It is important that both partners are willing participants of romantic overtures. "May I kiss you" whispered into the ear of one's romantic interest is very tender and sweet.
5. Keep the conversation light! Not everything has to be serious!
6. Shower your children with unconditional hugs and kisses.

Happy Kisses From Me to You!

———————

Be Real, Be You, Be Awesome this Holiday Season

The holiday season has snuck up on us once again. Scrambling to plan, shop, wrap, bake, cook, and party with friends leaves little time for us to pause and reflect on the past year. Therefore, let us skip that part of the New Year transition and focus on other topics, such as…your awesomeness as a parent.

Rather than offer "Ten Ways to Telepathically Communicate with your Child About Sex," the objective of today's piece is to focus on one's awesomeness as parents/caregivers. Consider this my holiday gift to you during this sometimes stressful season, despite it being the season of Peace and Love.

Mommy Manuals and Daddy Diaries

It is not that there are no Mommy Manuals or Daddy Diaries to assist us on our parenting journey; there are *many* manuals to guide parenting. You are reading one resource now, in fact. How do you choose which to read and how does one have time to read all those manuals AND have time to drink wine with friends? Priorities, right?

A friend once told me, "I have all the parenting books. I just don't have time to read them. I just want someone to tell me what to do." All my friends reading this are going to think I am quoting them. I am certain we have all muttered these words ourselves.

Here is where **your awesomeness** comes in: Merely by asking questions, talking to friends, and reading summaries in parenting book jackets, you are reaching out and gathering snippets of information to allow you to adapt the gazillion parenting suggestions into ideas that make sense for your family. Trying to parent without resources-human or otherwise-is lonely. Drinking wine with friends while bitching is a common social activity among women. A little wine with a little whine will often lead to some creative parenting suggestions.

The days of June Cleaver are history.

Your house is messy. Personally, I think it is perfectly normal to have a messy home. Your clean, but unkempt home, represents one (or two) of these scenarios:

a. You are spending time with your child in deep conversation about decision-making, future goals, values, and the state of the world.
b. You are (somewhat) mindlessly watching TV or a movie with your adolescent and mentally noting the potential conversation-starters featured in the current pop culture hit. (What? Sex without a condom!? Time for a conversation!)
c. You are relaxing and reading a book. And drinking wine. Always wine. Or beer. There's that, too.
d. You are too dang tired after working all day, chasing kids, volunteering, or being awesome-fill in the blank with your excuse... I mean reason.
e. Your child is scheduled to wash dishes on this particular evening but is nowhere to be seen.
f. You do not want to wash dishes right now. Plain and simple.

This is what makes **you awesome**: You realize the dishes are not going anywhere. They will be patiently waiting for you or another family member to wash them...later. One day, as you soak your dentures before bed and reflect upon your youthful decades as a parent, will it matter how efficient you were with the household chores? You are teaching your child that sometimes it is okay to slack off a little and just relax. Our society is so focused on doing, doing, doing to achieve some sort of perfection. Stress, anyone? Of course, if a messy house is what causes you stress, forget everything I just said and go wash your dishes while enjoying some wine.

Comfort Clothes

You run your errands in work out clothes. I totally do this. I work out early in the morning, so while I am in town I try to conserve my time and nature's resources (i.e. save money on gas), and get things done before heading home. By lunch, or even mid-morning, I begin to realize my attire should have morphed into "real" clothes by this point in the day. But hey, I'm in *work-out clothes*. I have a *reason* to look like this. In fact, sometimes I just wear workout clothes to run errands so I do not have to shower, deal with my hair, or wear make-up. Who will know the truth? I know I am not alone in this-I see men and women wearing running gear while running errands all the time.

And to those of us who do: **you are awesome**. You are communicating to the world that you value the benefits of healthy living (as you hide the package of candy bars under the quinoa in the grocery cart). You are communicating to your children that a person does not have to be dressed in the best clothes or wear lots of make-up to feel good about themselves. Their self-worth and self-esteem are based on who they are as a person, how they treat others, and their values. Naturally, our children do not need make-up and the best clothes-they inherited their good looks from their parents. We are awesome example-givers.

However, there is a balance. Our children do need to understand that how we present ourselves to the world is a reflection of how we view ourselves on the inside. Our children also need to be aware the workout clothes can only be used as an excuse occasionally. Presenting ourselves to the world in clean, neat clothes-and maybe with a dash of pizzazz-communicates confidence and self-respect. So, go be your awesome self in your sweats occasionally, but you have permission to splurge a little on something nice to wear. After all, it is for the kid's sake!

Yes, you are a perfect parent-because of your imperfection.

You are not a perfect parent, which is what makes you perfect. Being around someone who exudes perfectionism is incredibly intimidating. Besides, I have a little secret: There is no such thing as a perfect marriage, mom, dad, caregiver, child, teacher, human. In fact, it is peoples' imperfections that make them perfect people. So, embrace your **awesome imperfections** while embracing the imperfections of others. People will want to gather around your awesome self and embrace your imperfect awesomeness.

Finally....

During this season of Peace and Love, what I wish for each and every parent is to be able to let go of the craziness of the season and actually feel the peace and love we try to exude.

You are awesome. You reach out to others to support and be supported while raising your children. You understand that sometimes a messy house is a sign of a lived-in and loved-in home. You understand that sometimes, if you want to get stuff done, you just gotta get it done-no matter what you are wearing. You understand you are beautiful because of who you are on in inside-but deserve to splurge a little to beauty-up the outside, too. Finally, you understand that your kids are not perfect. Okay, neither are adults. Take time to sit back, block your view of dirty dishes, cuddle up and enjoy a fun Christmas/Holiday movie with your children while in your comfy leggings, and enjoy a glass of wine, beer, or cup of hot cocoa. With marshmallows. In other words, enjoy the magic of the season and pass that magic on to your kids.

THE MAGIC WILL BE AWESOMELY PERFECT.

The Gift of Time

Oh, boy. The kids are asked "what do you want for Christmas?" (or Hanukkah or whatever you may celebrate…even a birthday! Doesn't matter, really.) This is the big question our kids get asked each year.

Well, in this world of pretty cool technology, instead of an "album" by their favorite rock star, they are asking for some Apple device or another in which to download their favorite songs from iTunes. Just a *tad* more expensive than the $10 albums we used to find under the tree. (Okay, I admit, I love the tech stuff, too…)

What if, during this crazy, busy season, you and your significant young person take some time together to "bond" over hot chocolate, lunch, a drive in the car, or on a wintry walk in the woods… whatever your child prefers. I have found that one of the best places to get kids (and husbands, for that matter) to open up is on a quiet walk in the woods. There is something about physical activity that brings out the closeness in people. (I am sure I read somewhere that this has been scientifically proven, but there is no way I could ever find that study…) Not everyone has a forest preserve in their backyard, but maybe there is a park nearby, or just the sidewalk in your neighborhood. If that is not an option, a cup of cocoa at the kitchen table, with your undivided attention, works quite well.

You can use this time to talk about the upcoming new year. What are their plans, hopes, dreams, thoughts, about the upcoming year. If your child is in high school, you can approach the subject of college. Do they want to go? Where? What are their academic interests? You may have dreams of them becoming a doctor, but they see art school in their future…This is not the time to tell them *your* thoughts, this is the time to *listen* to *theirs*. Heaven knows we let them know exactly what we are thinking much of the time! (Your room is a mess! You didn't clear your plate! You didn't walk the dog!) Remember, this is their life journey to walk. We are merely here to give birth, feed, house, and pay for all the stuff they need to become decent adults in this world. And to be emotionally supportive of them, as well.

So, why am I encouraging this? Talking about sex and relationships with your child/grandchild/niece/nephew can be very difficult. By building a respectful relationship you are able to build trust with your child. And once you have trust, it will be easier for a deeper and more personal conversation to take place at a later time.

Take advantage of this magical holiday season. Take a walk and see some Christmas lights, stomp through the snow, walk on the beach (if you live somewhere warm, you lucky duck!)...and just enjoy the moment. In fact, I challenge parents to make this a regular event, not only around the holidays.

Disclaimer: You may see the "rolling of the eyeballs" on occasion during these peaceful, meaningful conversations. Don't take it personally. It merely means you are the smartest adult in the world, the young person just doesn't realize it yet. When they are college age they usually realize that you aren't as dumb as they thought. But of course by then, you realize that your kid does indeed know more than you in many, many aspects, like technology, science, and math. Don't let it get you down. Remember that once-upon-a-time, you knew how to add double-digits before they did.

Parents and Children: Learning Together

"But kids don't stay with you if you do it right. It's the one job where, the better you are, the more surely you won't be needed in the long run."— Barbara Kingsolver

As I write this, I have to laugh. I wonder if readers think I've raised these amazing, perfect daughters with absolutely no issues to deal with. Well, they are certainly amazing–as are YOUR children–and perfect–at least a perfect fit in our family–but no issues? Yeah, right.

Just know that there is no such thing as perfect parenting. We are all going to say something stupid, or hurtful, or wrong, or negative...or whatever it is your kid *says* you say that is wrong. (How many times do you hear "stop yelling at me!" when you are doing anything but yelling? In fact, you are merely biting your tongue?) And just *wait* till you start talking about s-e-x with them!

Feel good that you are doing the best you can with what you know and with whatever circumstance you are dealing with. If you blow it, like I have been known to do on many occasions, you can remedy it. Take a deep breath, calmly approach your teen and merely apologize.

Personally, I believe in letting them see the human side of you–you aren't just a dad or mom, you are a person. (I think they forget sometimes...) They will learn the awkward art of apologizing–and learn how to be a gracious forgiver. The benefits will come much later when they say something stupid, hurtful, or wrong to you and then follow-up with an apology. I can tell you from experience, there is nothing that melts your heart like being on the receiving end of a sincere apology from your child.

"The best way to keep children at home is to make the home atmosphere pleasant, and let the air out of the tires." — Dorothy Parker

---

Kim T. Cook, RN CHES

ADDITIONAL RESOURCES:

because you can't know everything

- AdvocatesforYouth.org
- aids.gov
- answer.rutgers.edu
- Centers for Disease Control and Prevention (CDC.gov)
- Future of Sex Education (futureofsexed.org)
- Guttmacher Institute (guttmacher.org)
- HealthyChildren.org
- heartwomenandgirls.org
- kidshealth.org
- Office of Adolescent Health (hhs.gov/ash/oah)
- Plannedparenthood.org
- pflag.org
- scarleteen.com
- SexEtc.org
- Sexuality Information and Education Council of the United States (SIECUS.org)
- suicidepreventionlifeline.org
- teenshealth.org
- teensource.org
- TeenWorldConfidential.com

Kim T. Cook, RN CHES

DISCLAIMER:

healthcare providers are your personal experts

Please remember – this information is not intended to be used to self-diagnose or replace any medical advice your healthcare provider will give you. It is only to inform and educate. Please see your healthcare provider if you have any questions, problems, symptoms, issues, and concerns regarding sexual health.

Kim T. Cook, RN CHES

ACKNOWLEDGMENTS:

i know some awesome people

One lazy, sunny Sunday afternoon while channeling a beached whale wallowing in the pool, I mentioned to my friend and confidant that I had kind of a crazy idea. I wanted to write a fiction book for young people using the National Sexuality Education Standards. I thought this would be a clever and unique educational tool for students to learn about sex, relationships, decison-making, and values. This close friend, Kristy Maher, enthusiastically encouraged me. She suggested I talk with Denise Dorman of WriteBrain Media. With Denise's help, Teen World Confidential was launched.

However, after writing the first sentence of my fiction book, I realized I did not like the daunting assignment I gave myself; it was an incredibly arduous five minutes! Because I am my own boss, I gave myself permission to regroup and try again. Hence, the book you are reading now.

There are many selfless people who have encouraged, supported, and advised me along this journey—and likely have no idea how impactful their kindness is. Jill Salzman of *The Founding Moms* taught me to follow my passion and listen to my inner entrepreneurial voice. Peter Himmelman of *Big Muse* encouraged me to acknowledge vulnerabilities, push through, and take a chance. Justin Ahrens of *Rule 29 Creative* gave his valuable time and expertise to encourage and educate when I felt particularly dazed. Beth Bannor patiently assists with my temperamental website.

Dr. Sally Conklin encouraged and supported my efforts from the first day we met at Northern Illinois University. Dr. Carolyn Mills happily offered her medical expertise. Ellie Sterner, my first intern, whose enthusiasm for this project made me realize early on that perhaps I'm on to something.

Julie Pheney, educator extraordinaire, taught me that perfection does not exist in the teaching world—you do your best, learn from it and move on. It was the first time I had been given permission to fail, and that failure is an important opportunity to grow. This allowed me to relax and enjoy my journey with a little less stress and pressure.

The students I have had the privilege of caring for, communicating with, and educating over the last couple of decades have taught me the importance of being **real**. Young people want an adult with whom they can talk honestly and openly about sex, without fear of judgment. My happiest work memories are the connections I made with the remarkable young people in the school community.

Professional organizations provide research and education to enable comprehensive, accurate information to be disseminated by educators like myself. Society for Public Health Education (SOPHE), American School Health Association (ASHA), Illinois School Health Education (ISHA), Society for Adolescent Health and Medicine (SAHM), American Academy of Pediatrics (AAP), Planned Parenthood, and individual professionals such as Nora Gelperin of Advocates for Youth and Lori Reichel, Ph.D deserve accolades for the work they are doing to ensure that young people get the education they need and deserve. Thank you for making my job that much easier.

A *special heartfelt thank you* to a tribe of friends who comment on my posts, send me relevant articles, offer quotes and suggestions, and allow me to blab on-and-on about "the book" that has taken forever to write: Katie Bartindale, Amy Storm, Rose Haeseli, Sue Bowman, Nancy Stanis, Dawn Joyce-Meier, and Aldona McBain are the core that keep me accountable and forward-moving. Hugs. Other friends who have contributed to my mental health by providing friendship and/or libations include libations include Kelly Kelley, Patty Bixler, Mary Sterner, Laura Macklin-Purdy, Luciene Moore, Donna Bode, Pam Smith, Lisa Conrath-Bova, Ivette Bolander, Karen and Tim Sheehan, Marcy Zirbel, Diane Sheppard, Joanna Duensing, Sue Melton, Mary Sunday, and my other lovely friends from bunco, book club, running, and workout. Thank you all for your encouragement and support.

My deepest appreciation to Tess Bondavalli who selflessly edited each and every one of one my pieces. Her daily reminders of the importance of the Teen World Confidential message keeps me moving forward—some days a little slower than others. I absolutely could not have done this without her. Tara Vanderheyden, a creative talent, offers a listening ear and innovative ideas when the need arises. 25N Coworking offered not only a quiet place to work, but thoughtful people with whom I was able to share ideas and receive helpful advice—thank you. Zack and Rob Price of *Blog to Book Publishing*-thank you for your patience and support.

And then there is my family. My parents—all kinds of parents—who love unconditionally: Andy VanderSloot, Millie VanderSloot, Pat Watson, Sandy Cook, Jim Cook, Joyce VanderMolen. (I miss you, Dad.) My nieces and nephews who are emerging adults and whose faces I see when I write. When Morgan the Great, Jack, Will, Ben, Austin, Tyler, or Hayden say, "Hey, Aunt Kim!"—my heart sings. My brothers Kent and Kevin VanderSloot and their families, and my friend Janey Cornett, whom I love like a sister, help me understand the richness of family relationships.

My husband Bob quietly sits by the sidelines while I follow my calling and forge this crazy path. He understands my passion and drive to make a difference in the lives of families and supports me unconditionally. My daughters Jennifer, Caitlin, and Molly taught me that being a parent is not easy, but it is—hands down—the best "job" I could ever dream of. My daughters inspire me each and every day to be the best person I can be. My family rocks—I am a lucky woman. I love you.

Finally, my mother, like so many women of her generation, is the bridge between generations past of women with limited opportunities to the dynamic, independent women of today. She has inspired me to teach my daughters what it means to be unfettered and bold. Whether my daughters choose to become homemakers, continue on their career paths, or something in between, the choice is theirs thanks to women of my mother's generation and the women who follow. Thanks, Mom.

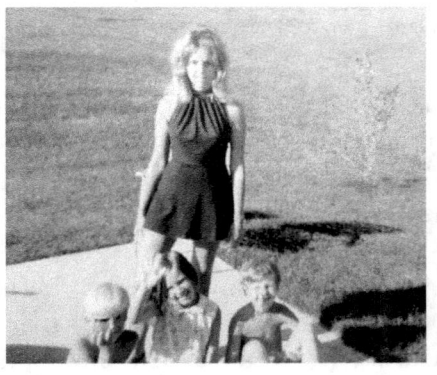

www.ingramcontent.com/pod-product-compliance
Lightning Source LLC
Chambersburg PA
CBHW071331280526
45787CB00001B/67